Supervision in Sp
Language Therapy

Supervision plays a central role in supporting professional practice, practitioner wellbeing, clinical governance and client safety. This anthology, designed as a collection of possibilities rather than a definitive guide, offers a window into a less visible and rarely discussed aspect of practice. Contributors draw on first-hand encounters of supervision to share insights from both professional and public perspectives. These span practice contexts from pre-registration to qualified and into advanced clinical practice and management roles. The accounts include individual, team, multi-professional, independent and public sector experiences within and beyond the speech and language therapy profession. This book:

- Broadens the discourse and deepens understanding about supervision theory and practice
- Explores multiple formats and contrasting approaches to lay bare differences in the enactment of supervision as well as variations in underlying assumptions and real-life supervision challenges
- Holds a mirror up to diverse conversations about supervision across practice contexts and career points to broaden the scope of supervision possibilities
- Prompts exploration of new ways to engage with and benefit from supervision as an alternative or adjunct to existing, established approaches
- Demonstrates the clear return on investment in supervision at personal, departmental, service and organisational levels with both professional and public benefit

Illustrated throughout with personal stories and professional wisdom, this book will interest students and practitioners at all stages of their career in speech and language therapy. In addition, it will appeal to other allied health and care professionals. This anthology aims to stimulate reflection on contemporary issues in supervision as well as individual, service and organisational supervision culture and practice.

Cathy Sparkes has been a champion for high quality supervision for many years, encompassing her working life as a speech and language therapist, personal construct psychology (PCP) counsellor and supervisor.

Sam Simpson, an independent speech and language therapist, person-centred counsellor, supervisor and trainer, plays an active role in teaching about supervision, promoting pro-supervision cultures and developing robust, quality supervision practices across the UK public and independent sectors.

Deborah Harding is a speech and language therapist by profession. She is Professor of Learning and Innovation for Practice at City St George's, University of London and has advisory roles with the National Health Service in England.

Supervision in Speech and Language Therapy

Personal Stories and Professional Wisdom

Edited by
Cathy Sparkes, Sam Simpson and Deborah Harding

Routledge
Taylor & Francis Group

LONDON AND NEW YORK

Designed cover image: © Getty Images

First published 2025
by Routledge
4 Park Square, Milton Park, Abingdon, Oxon OX14 4RN

and by Routledge
605 Third Avenue, New York, NY 10158

Routledge is an imprint of the Taylor & Francis Group, an informa business

British Library Cataloguing-in-Publication Data
A catalogue record for this book is available from the British Library

ISBN: 978-1-032-29341-7 (hbk)
ISBN: 978-1-032-29342-4 (pbk)
ISBN: 978-1-003-30114-1 (ebk)

DOI: 10.4324/9781003301141

Typeset in Optima
by Apex CoVantage, LLC

Contents

Contents

Acknowledgements

This book is the product of enormous collective effort.

First, we are hugely grateful to the chapter authors who found time to share their stories and wisdom, and who remained committed to the vision of this publication during unanticipated life transitions and wider global challenges. We would also like to thank both Jane Madeley and Molly Kavanagh at Taylor and Francis for their guidance, encouragement and flexibility throughout the journey to publication. Additionally, we appreciate everyone who granted permission to reproduce figures and diagrams for inclusion herein.

Importantly, we would like to acknowledge all the colleagues, practitioners and students plus all the supervisors and supervisees who we have worked with over the years. These valuable relationships and experiences have facilitated our varied and diverse paths to this point and fuelled our commitment to support robust supervision theory and practice. We hope that through this anthology our own personal and professional insights and perspectives provide a healthy mix of clarity and challenge, resulting in a rich and engaging exploration of supervision in its many forms.

Professionally, we would each like to acknowledge specific influences in our own supervision narratives. Cathy would especially like to thank her first supervisor Peggy Dalton, who showed her the way and Mary Frances, longstanding coach and inspiration. Sam is grateful for the cumulative fingerprints all her supervisors, supervisees, co-facilitators and course participants have left on her supervision practice. They have enabled her to keep learning. Deborah would like to acknowledge how recent experiences with policy and decision-making colleagues have challenged her go-to assumptions and solutions.

At a personal level, we are each grateful for the support and encouragement of our partners, families and friends who sustained us throughout this project.

Finally, we would like to acknowledge that it is because we are all ordinary people, reliant on the compassion and skill of others in our most vulnerable moments, that investing in regular, effective and thoughtful supervision really matters.

Contributors

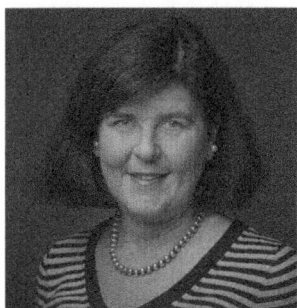

Ann Farquhar has been a practicing speech and language therapist for over 30 years in charitable, NHS and independent contexts and currently is a clinical tutor at City, University of London. She has maintained her curiosity between the links across different client groups: working with children and teenagers with language and social communication needs in schools and an interest in children and adults with acquired brain injury. Ann's independent practice offers supervision services for colleagues.

Cathy Sparkes works as a personal construct psychology (PCP) counsellor and supervisor. She originally worked as a speech and language therapist (SLT) with individuals who had experienced a neurological condition and their support networks. Since 2003 she has worked as a counsellor with this same client group. Cathy has extensive experience of receiving and providing supervision and has been a champion for high quality supervision practice for many years.

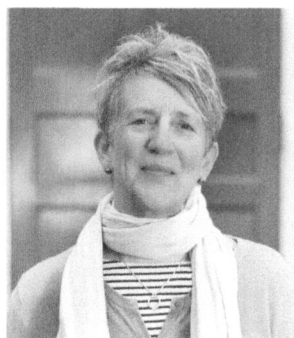

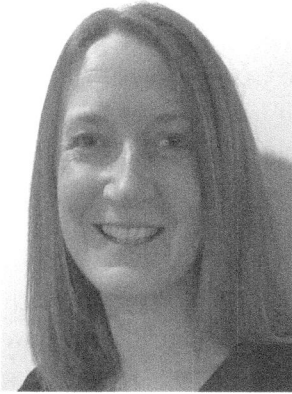

Claire Farrington-Douglas is a speech and language therapist working in the field of acquired brain injury and dementia. She specialises in group interventions, communication partner training and delivering intensive comprehensive aphasia programmes (ICAPs). She is passionate about involving family and friends in interventions to ensure therapy is meaningful. Claire works as an external supervisor and is continually developing her supervision practice in creative ways.

Dawn Leoni is currently a service manager within NHS Wales. She has been a practicing speech and language therapist for 25 years, working clinically within adult services. She has worked in a range of NHS, private and public sector organisations in England and Wales, and continues to advocate for excellence in therapy practices.

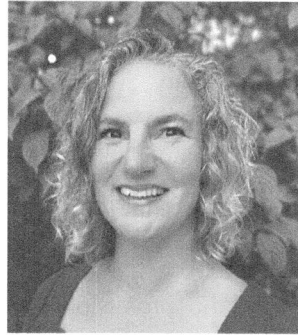

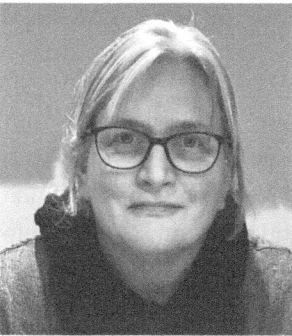

Deborah Harding is a speech and language therapist by profession. She combines her role as Professor of Learning and Innovation for Practice at City St George's, University of London with work developing national guidance for the National Health Service in England and beyond. Her teaching, research and policy work are underpinned by her comprehensive experience in multi-professional health and social care practice, management and leadership. Deborah's PhD research explored supervision for the allied health professions.

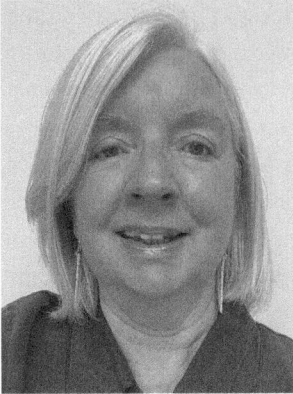

Edel O'Dea has worked as a speech and language therapist in Ireland for over 40 years, mostly in the public health service. She has learned valuable life lessons in her quest to understand the complex lived experience of stammering. Edel is currently involved in education and advocacy and is a founding member of the Irish Stammering Association's *Brod Staidearachta* (Stammering Pride) group which gently invites others to join in exploring how to dismantle barriers and create a culture that embraces stammering voices.

Fran Brander is a consultant physiotherapist at the National Hospital for Neurology & Neurosurgery. She has always worked within the National Health Service, specialising in complex inpatient and stroke rehabilitation, with a special interest in upper limb rehabilitation. Fran has a strong commitment to evidence-based practice and is passionate about the professional development of her team and the wider profession as a whole, through teaching and supervision.

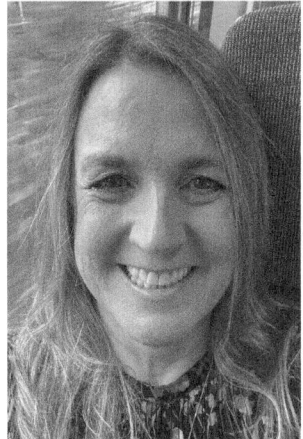

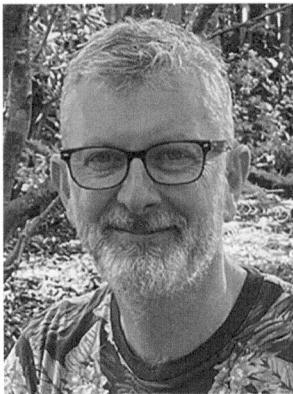

Gavin Newby is an experienced consultant clinical neuropsychologist working with acquired brain injury. His career has spanned both the NHS and independent sector. Gavin has provided, and received, individual and group supervision. He is informed by an eclectic approach to supervision but has a particular interest in Personal Constructs and Systemic therapy frameworks.

Iain Wilkie is the founder of the international charity 50 Million Voices for adults who stammer and for employers interested in unleashing the terrific potential of stammering talent. A former senior partner with EY, he is also an accredited executive coach and mentor specialising in helping quieter leaders and executives with disabilities to thrive in a working world designed by extroverts and ableists. The World Stuttering & Cluttering Organisation (WSCO) recognised Iain's work with their 2024 award for the 'Individual who improved the lives of people who stutter and clutter' and for his 'unique contribution to the community of people who stutter'. Iain enjoys Americana music and singing, while also relishing spending time outdoors surrounded by nature.

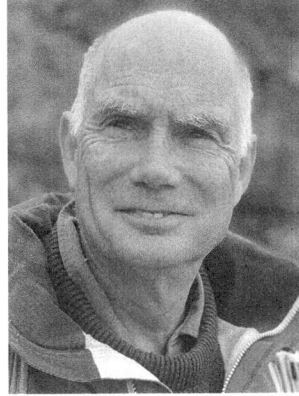

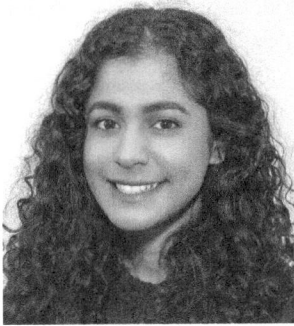

Ilyeh Nahdi is a highly specialist speech and language therapist with experience in predominantly community paediatric settings. She has been termed a "trailblazer" in promoting diversity within the profession. As the co-creator of SLTea Time, a pioneering platform fostering dialogue on the ethnic minority experience in speech and language therapy, Ilyeh has garnered recognition, earning accolades such as the NHS Emerging Leader award for outstanding EDI contributions. A 2021 graduate of the Future Leaders Programme, she served on the Royal College of Speech and Language Therapists (RCSLT) board of trustee's Nomination Panel committee. Ilyeh continues to work alongside the RCSLT in actively shaping the future of the field through collaborative efforts on EDI, policies, and service development projects.

Jackie McRae completed her training as a speech and language therapist in London in 1991 and after a brief period working with children, her clinical focus has been with adults with acquired complex speech and swallowing difficulties in the intensive care setting. As this has been an evolving area of speciality, she has developed new services and supervised many clinicians to ensure best practice. This has informed her research on the effective clinical management of people with spinal cord injury.

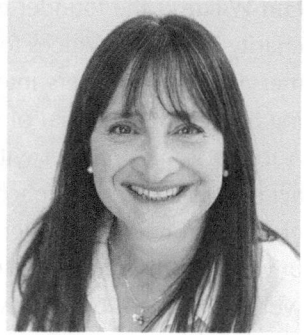

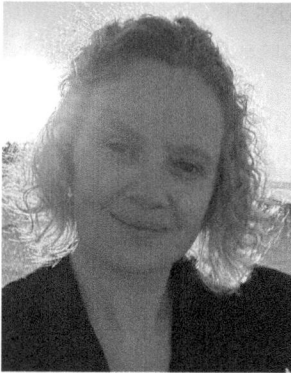

Jennifer Roche has been an NHS speech and language therapist since 2005 and currently works as the clinical lead for stammering in Oldham, Greater Manchester. Jen is a senior lecturer at Manchester Metropolitan University, where she supervises stammering research, and has held clinical leadership positions in the independent sector and has worked with the voluntary sector.

Justin Roe is a Consultant and Professional Lead for Speech and Language Therapy at the Royal Marsden NHS Foundation Trust (RM) in London. In addition to his clinical work, he leads on multidisciplinary rehabilitation service provision to people receiving treatment from head and neck, lung cancers and neuro-oncology services at the Marsden. He is also leads the complex laryngology/ airway reconstruction service at Imperial College Healthcare NHS Trust. He is a Professor of Practice in Speech and Swallowing Rehabilitation in the Department of Surgery and Cancer at Imperial College London.

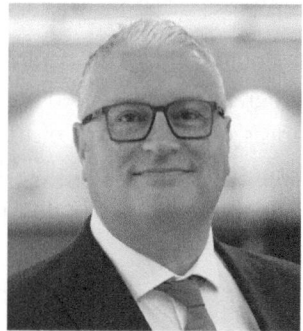

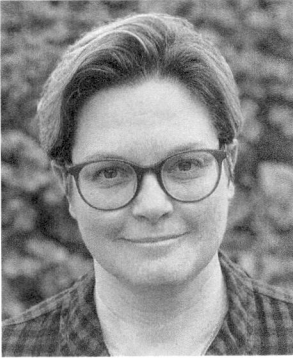

Karen Cundy has been a speech and language therapist for 17 years, with a specialist interest in working alongside children and adults with acquired brain injury and autism. Karen has worked in a wide range of settings, including acute, residential and community neurorehabilitation within the NHS, and specialist and mainstream schools. Her independent practice also offers professional supervision services for MDT professionals and speech and language therapy practitioners.

Kate Ashforth is the Professional Lead for speech and language therapy at the Royal Marsden NHS Foundation Trust in London. As Associate Lead she also manages a range of allied health professionals in a variety of professions, who provide multidisciplinary rehabilitation, across the pathway. Kate was the co-founder of the Royal College of Speech and Language Therapists (RCSLT) Head and Neck Clinical Excellence Network South, and she contributes to work for the RCSLT and NHS England. Kate was awarded the Fellowship of the RCSLT in recognition of her contribution and advancement of the profession.

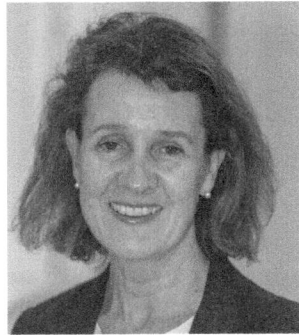

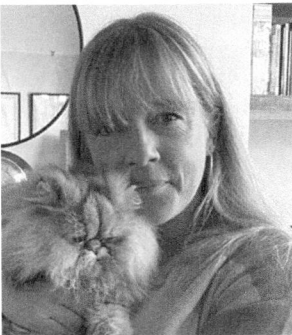

Kate Balzer has worked with adults since qualifying as a speech and language therapist from UCL in 1999, mainly with acquired neurological conditions but also mental health difficulties. Following the birth of her daughters and service restructures, she moved from Principal SLT in the NHS to independent practice. Currently, she enjoys a portfolio of roles, as a treating therapist in medico legal cases, providing clinical cover for care homes and facilitating project groups for adults with cognitive communication disorders.

Kimerley Clarke has worked as a speech and language therapist/speech pathologist for over 32 years in both clinical and leadership roles in Australia and the United Kingdom. Kim has been a professional advisor for a number of professional body guidelines and position papers. Since 2017, she has been in private practice providing clinical services with adults and professional supervision via video-conferencing.

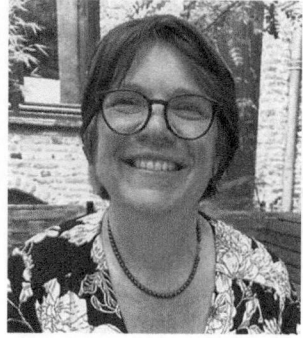

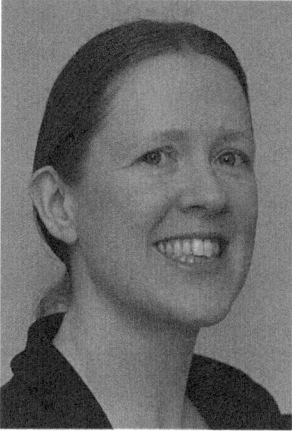

Lauren Tyson (*née* Wright) is an independent speech and language therapist based in West Sussex and draws inspiration from her father's stammering journey. With a background in the NHS, she is the owner of That Speech Lady. Lauren successfully led an innovative outdoor group for children who stammer, and her collaboration with Gareth Gates further enriched her perspective. She supports individuals of all ages, aiming to reshape societal perceptions of stammering and embrace the unique differences in speech.

Lorraine Maher-Edwards is a registered specialist practitioner psychologist. She is an experienced clinician, researcher, supervisor, and trainer with a particular interest in Acceptance and Commitment Therapy, Compassion Focused Therapy and Mindfulness Based Cognitive Therapy. At present, Lorraine splits her time between a senior role in a busy NHS oncology team in London and her private practice. Lorraine identifies as someone who experiences stammering. She was involved in the NHS Stammering Network and has mentored people who stammer.

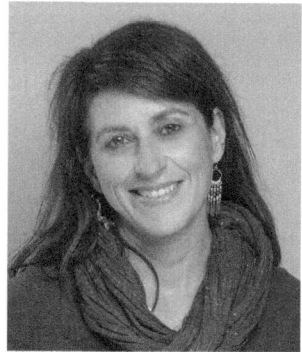

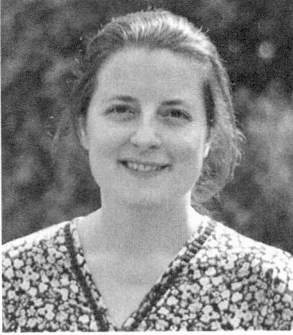

Lucie Rochfort is currently Course Leader and Lecturer for the MSc Speech and Language Therapy (pre-registration) course at AECC University College in Bournemouth, developing the next generation of competent evidence-based speech and language therapists. She is an HCPC registered speech and language therapist and a member of the RCSLT, with experience of working in both the NHS and private sector, specialising in acquired brain injury rehabilitation. She has particular interest in healthcare leadership, coaching and supervision.

Lucy Titheridge is now an advanced clinical practitioner (ACP) in Derby. Lucy works clinically in Geriatrics, but has been fortunate to rotate and work in a variety of medical specialities, since starting her training in 2017. More recently she has moved into medical education working with medical students along with her clinical work as an ACP. She regularly supervises medical students during their last three years of medical school. Having worked as a speech and language therapist for 13 years in the field of adult care, including stroke and Ear, Nose and Throat (ENT), she made the transition into advanced clinical practice to broaden her knowledge, skills and job role to be able work with more advanced clinical skills but maintain her SLT background and bring that dimension to the ACP role.

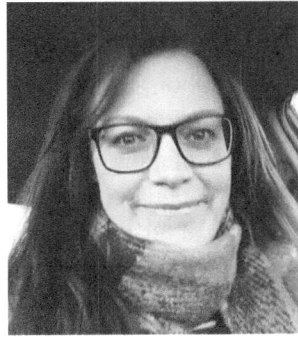

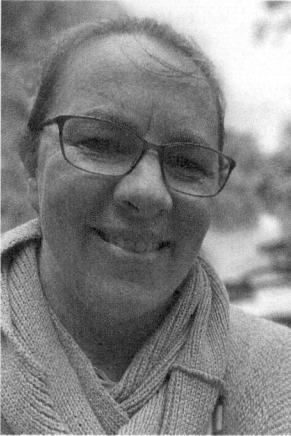

Mary Ganpatsingh worked in the NHS and charity sector before setting up her independent speech and language practice in 2009, working with adults who have acquired brain injury. She specialises in working with people experiencing complex, cognitive communication difficulties, particularly where these impact real-life roles and relationships. Mary increasingly delivers therapy in real-life settings, such as workplaces and leisure facilities. She is also a professional supervisor and is developing an interest in writing and speaking about her work.

Melanie Cross is a speech and language therapist, author, trainer and Video Interaction Guidance supervisor. Her work has focused on increasing awareness of the links between speech, language and communication needs and mental health challenges in young people as well as developing speech and language therapy services for children and young people with Social Emotional and Mental Health needs (SEMH).

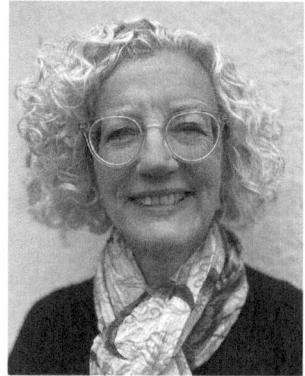

Melanie Packer qualified as a speech and language therapist in 2006. Melanie joined Birmingham City University in 2018 and is now a Senior Lecturer. Up until March 2024 she had a strategic overview for speech and language therapy placements. Melanie is now the BSc Hons Speech and Language Therapy Course Lead. Melanie is currently completing a professional doctorate and maintains special interests in professional practice, innovation in practice-based learning and the development of a diverse workforce.

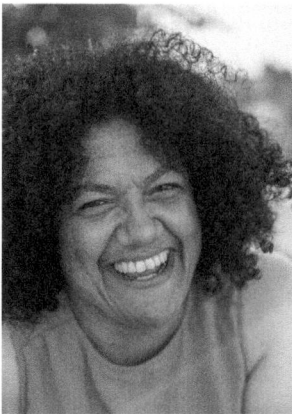

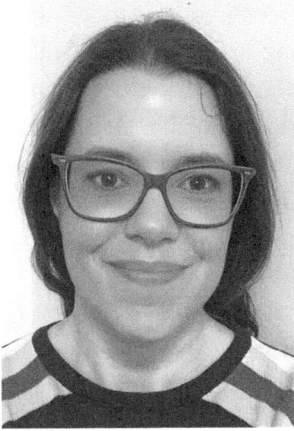

Penny Farrell qualified as a speech and language therapist in Wales in 2002 and currently works in independent practice in Ireland. Additionally, Penny is a clinical practice educator with speech and language therapy students and the Youth Development Officer with the Irish Stammering Association (ISA). Penny is one of the founder members of the ISA *Brod Staidearachta* (Stammering Pride) group and also contributed to Conor Foran's *Dysfluent* magazine (Issue 2, 2023) on the celebrations and challenges of Stammering Pride.

Rachel Barton has worked as a speech and language therapist for almost 30 years. After 22 years as a paediatric therapist in the NHS Rachel left the safety of an employed role to set up her own independent practice. Over the past six years, alongside developing a clinical service to local families and schools, Rachel has built a successful supervision service supporting speech and language therapists throughout the UK.

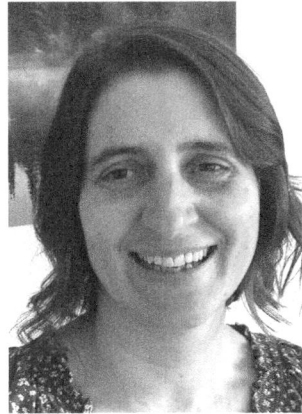

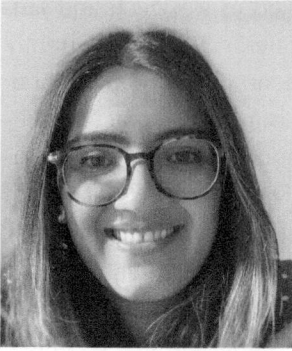

Sahar Nashir is a speech and language therapist (SLT) specialising in Paediatric Acquired Brain Injury within the NHS. She is currently working in the United Arab Emirates as a SLT in a multidisciplinary team, supporting children and families. Sahar is the daughter of Afghan-diaspora living in the United Kingdom. She has a background in psychology and teaching, and has a particular interest in understanding and reducing the inequalities that exist in healthcare systems. Within the last few years, she has had the privilege of engaging with Anti-Racism work with peers as part of 'SLTea Time' and wider collaborations across the SLT profession. Outside of clinical practice and writing, Sahar finds peace in being outdoors, self-care and travelling.

Sam Simpson is an independent speech and language therapist, person-centred counsellor, supervisor and trainer. She is a committed supervisee and holds a Diploma in Person Centred Supervision from Metanoia Institute to ground her work as a supervisor. Sam enjoys supervising across specialisms and professions, valuing the intimacy of 1:1 working and the collaborative learning of paired and group supervision. Sam plays an active role in teaching about supervision, promoting pro-supervision cultures and developing robust, quality supervision practices across the UK public and independent sectors.

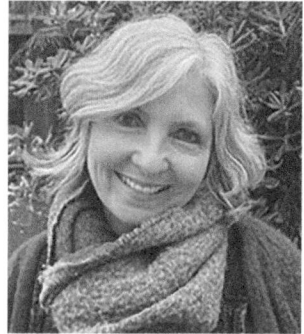

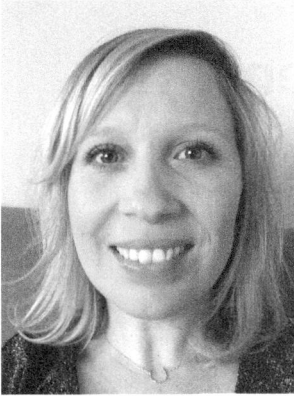

Sarah Stewart has worked as a speech and language therapist for over 20 years specialising in acquired brain injury. She has worked in the National Health Service as clinical lead across the neurosciences pathway and is currently in independent practice in the community in East Sussex. Sarah also works as a clinical tutor at University College London supporting the future speech and language therapy workforce. Sarah is passionate about supervision and all it can bring to the individual, the profession and to the client.

Scott Ballard-Ridley is a qualified physiotherapist. Not long after graduating, Scott suffered a major stroke which left him with significant physical impairments, including the complete loss of his vision. Scott has worked in NHS Stroke services and for the Stroke Association. Since 2016, he has worked for the social enterprise Bridges Self-Management to support healthcare practitioners in practice and research to adopt a more person-

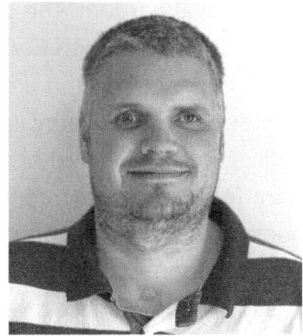

alised approach to their work. Since 2020, Scott has also worked with NHS England to explore ways of bringing more lived experience to the development of policy.

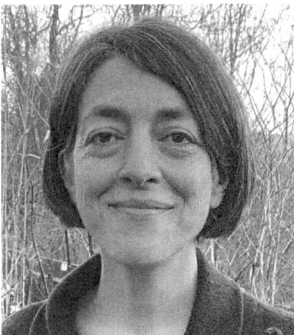

Zein Pereira is a speech and language therapist with over 30 years' experience. Following 11 years as a clinical lead in the NHS, she worked for the parent charity, Afasic. Zein currently works independently, offering speech and language therapy, professional supervision, training, and mentoring. Zein enjoys collaborating with children, families, and colleagues, to enable a resourceful approach to supporting development and change.

Introduction

Cathy Sparkes, Sam Simpson and Deborah Harding

Welcome to this supervision anthology: a collection of personal stories and professional wisdom. The opportunity to create this publication arose when Routledge approached Cathy with a request to address a gap they had identified in the supervision literature for the speech and language therapy (SLT) profession. In turn Cathy approached both Sam and Deborah, longstanding colleagues who shared her background in SLT and enthusiasm for supervision. Together we formed an editorial team and discussion began about the book we wanted to craft. We quickly agreed we did not want to produce a how-to book. Instead, drawing on our knowledge, skills and experience of supervision practices, we were keen to gather and share contrasting personal accounts which would illustrate the rich diversity of the supervision landscape.

As editors, each of our supervision perspectives have been developed through our own experiences of supervision as supervisees and supervisors as well as training, reading, teaching, researching, professional networks and role models. Collectively, we bring experience in SLT, counselling, coaching, leadership and academia. We draw on diverse frameworks and theoretical positions, including personal construct psychology, person centred therapy, practitioner permeability and action learning. We are committed to and in some instances have influenced national, professional body and regulatory policy and guidance, including the Royal College of Speech and Language Therapists (RCSLT), Association of Speech and Language Therapists in Independent Practice (ASLTIP), Health and Care Professions Council (HCPC), United Kingdom Council for Psychotherapy (UKCP), British Association of Counselling and Psychotherapy (BACP) and the National Health Service (NHS) England Centre for Advancing Practice. Collectively, we have

110 years of practice experience spanning five decades during which we have seen a welcome evolution in supervision practice and accompanying guidance.

The initial brief for the book focused on supervision practice within the SLT profession. Most contributors are anchored in SLT, however, some extend beyond this scope, providing a balance of personal and professional insights. As editors we drew on personal and professional relationships and connections to bring together perspectives from different contexts. Authors include those with lived experiences of using SLT services alongside a multi-professional mix of supervisee, supervisor, practitioner, manager, educator and academic voices. The result is an eclectic collection of insights, predominantly but not exclusively from the United Kingdom public and private health, care and education sectors.

The stories gathered here bring supervision into the public domain in ways we hope you will find vibrant and engaging. They capture the richness, complexity and diversity of supervision. The sharing of different lived experiences of supervision affirms its value and potential for individual clients and practitioners as well as wider organisations and systems. We are reminded of the need to be aware of a possible spectrum of supervision cultures and practices and that our taken-for-granted assumptions may not be the same as those of our colleagues. As a minimum, it highlights the need for open dialogue about our experiences, understandings and expectations of supervision and the extent to which these are articulated, negotiated and aligned.

As editors, each of us has brought our individual constellation of experiences of professional practice and supervision. An eye-opening aspect of the editorial process has been the exposure of some fundamental differences in our own supervision beliefs and approaches. These have been greater in number than we might have predicted or anticipated and navigating this has not been without challenge and debate. We share this to illustrate that even with richly elaborated views about supervision, we have benefited from open dialogue regarding these similarities and differences. Our discussions have highlighted that we each have our go-to anchors born out of our unique lived experiences, theoretical lenses and research perspectives. We have realised that even though we have invested a good deal of our professional selves in supervision there is an ongoing need to pay attention to our own assumptions in this field. This perhaps reflects the supervisory relationship and the need to review this regularly as practitioner experience and understanding evolves over time. Furthermore, it reinforces the importance of 'supervision *of* supervision' as a way to identify possible blind spots.

Our hope is that this anthology gives you the opportunity to reflect on your own supervision history, current practice and to explore future alternatives. The range and variety of stories reflects the varied landscape of supervision practice. This book offers a window into an aspect of practice which is deeply personal, private and rarely discussed. You will see that the diversity of the SLT profession and the contexts in which speech and language therapists work, both established and emerging, are reflected in the experiences of supervision captured in each chapter. By exploring multiple formats and contrasting approaches, the book lays bare differences in the enactment of supervision to reveal variations in underlying assumptions and understandings. Supervision is a developing field with a broad evolution of ideas emerging. We aim to hold a mirror up to diverse conversations about supervision across different practice influences. We are reminded of the importance of regularly checking in with one another about our own experiences, expectations and perspectives.

We asked our contributors to provide a combination of personal stories and professional wisdom. As we expected, each author has their own prism through which they construe supervision. Whilst the balance of personal story and professional wisdom varies from chapter to chapter, multiple viewpoints are represented. As we take stock, a number of recurrent themes have emerged:

Influence of different practice contexts

Our book shares insights about supervision practice from professional and public standpoints. These span clinical and practice contexts from pre-registration to qualified and into advanced clinical practice and management roles. The accounts draw on individual, team, multi-professional, independent and public sector experiences across specialisms, such as children and young people, oncology, stammering, critical care and acquired brain injury.

Our contributors explore supervision from diverse backgrounds and identities, differing levels of experience and from within practice and beyond. We feel that the chapters bring to life the many and varied practice landscapes that speech and language therapists work in and we see there is a strong sense of energy, voice and commitment to supervision throughout.

The chapters illustrate how practitioners consider similar and different approaches to supervision across practice settings and career points. We hope this variety will prompt exploration of new ways to experiment, engage with and benefit from supervision alongside or to augment existing, familiar approaches.

Definitions of supervision

Across the chapters there are different interpretations and definitions of supervision which in turn influence practice. Each chapter demonstrates the possibility of supervision rather than offering a definitive position. Some authors use supervision as a 'catch all' term, an umbrella for a range of interpretations and activities, whereas others seek to establish a more refined or clearly differentiated understanding. Learning about supervision is a dynamic, ongoing endeavour. The difference in terms of language use and the boundaries of the terms assigned and the activities they depict is an ongoing conversation within and across professions. This highlights the importance of regularly revisiting how the word supervision is used and applied.

In the literature there are different uses of language, perspective and emphasis when defining supervision theory and practice. We have encouraged authors to be explicit and consistent in their preferred definitions and terminology and to explore for themselves any ambiguity these may reveal. Across the chapters, the word supervision is used much of the time to refer to a sacred, confidential, boundaried space with a mutually agreed purpose. It is a space where there are relational considerations, shared understanding and negotiated dialogue regarding the principles and dimensions of supervision, formalised by a contract or working agreement. The chapters have prompted us to consider the extent to which the term supervision might encompass other professional development activities. In particular to explore which dimensions of professional learning, development, wellbeing and reflection sit under the term supervision. As editors and practitioners, we notice that one way in which the supervisory purpose is differentiated is to apply a qualifying adjective to supervision, such as professional, managerial, clinical, educational. Additionally, some authors have differentiated supervision which takes place privately and *away* from practice from supervision that takes place *in* a practice or clinical setting. We have hotly debated different terminology, our associated understandings and the activities they signify. Examples include *in* supervision (in a sacred space), *under* supervision (in a practice context) and the difference between supervision *in-action* and *on-action*. We know that contracting can help to ensure that all supervisory relationships are clear regarding the differences between supervision, education, counselling and governance. Crucially, we are reminded of the value of finding a supervisory match for the supervisee's needs in terms of both supervisor and supervisory approach and purpose, as well as regularly reviewing individual experiences, expectations and associated understandings.

Standards

In many chapters the relationship between supervision, standards, legislation and professional regulation is acknowledged. Throughout our own careers we have witnessed the strengthening status of supervision as fundamental to robust, quality practice. In organisations where a culture of supervision is established, this can have a positive impact on practitioner recruitment, retention, psychological safety and development. Some chapters refer to professional bodies and regulators, such as the Royal College of Speech and Language Therapists and the Health and Care Professions Council, which set out member and registrant responsibilities for active participation in supervision. Other chapters highlight the growing awareness across employers of their legal responsibilities to ensure the availability of supervision and the associated links to public safety. Guidance and standards within supervision are essential in order to keep practitioners and clients safe but also to offer a platform for dialogue and negotiation at individual, team, service and organisational levels.

We would welcome a more robust stance from regulators and professional bodies in relation to supervision. The extent to which adherence to existing regulatory standards and legislative mandates are specifically interrogated at points of registrant renewal and employer inspection is unknown. What might strengthen the imperative for tighter scrutiny would be focused research to demonstrate the valuable relationship between supervision, professional safety, wellbeing and public safety. Arguably without a rigorous evidence base, it is difficult for regulatory or inspection bodies to be more emphatic about supervision as an imperative for practitioners or employers, and limits progress towards developing more definitive standards.

Establishing cultural norms

Many of the chapters reference directly or indirectly the importance and value of early and continuous education about supervision. Contributors refer to the absence of supervision theory in SLT training and the need for training to support greater theory into practice and a more elaborate understanding of supervision. Several chapters plot the process of coming to understand the value of supervision. For some contributors this awareness prompts engagement in training. For others, engagement in training serves as an epiphany about supervision and a catalyst for further development, experimentation and discovery. There are striking examples of the ways in which supervision-focused professional development has prompted the critical appraisal of taken-for-granted assumptions about supervision and sparked a re-evaluation of the similarities and differences between professional support and supervision. The wisdom shared in this book includes awakenings about developing as a supervisee and supervisor being a necessary continuing professional development (CPD) consideration. Drawing on our professional experiences, we observe that from early career and beyond, practitioners tend to focus their CPD on clinical knowledge and skills. The result is a neglect of other fundamental aspects of practice and a default position that mistakenly assumes effective supervision is achieved through vicarious learning alone. Several chapters support this observation and demonstrate the value of expanding CPD beyond clinical practice to include ongoing development in supervision.

We notice those who become skilful supervisees and supervisors have invested in their development specifically around supervision. Across the chapters there are examples of this development in relation to reflective practice, facilitation, psychological safety and counselling skills. Insightful supervisors recognise the need to hone their own supervision knowledge and skills. They proactively engage in supervisor training, accessing a range of supervision learning opportunities and ensure regular supervision *of* supervision. They recognise the need for ongoing learning opportunities to keep their supervision practice fresh, alive and creative. Interestingly, these observations do not seem to be unique to speech and language therapists as the contributors from outside of SLT indicate similar awakenings and insights.

This is not a book about becoming a supervisee nor developing supervisors. However, there are indicators throughout showing the importance of ongoing growth and development as both supervisees and supervisors. It is evident the contributors have learned in different, healthy and helpful ways, through interweaving themes of training, experience and experimentation within and across their respective careers and professional journeys. What we can see from our authors is that without good foundations in what supervision is and is not, supervision practice invariably becomes a mirror of supervision received where there is a risk of perpetuating poor practice.

Organisational culture

Leadership and organisational values can influence and shape supervision culture. Some chapters focus specifically on developing pro-supervision organisational cultures. Others highlight how organisational factors influence supervision. This is illustrated through examples of cultures which actively promote supervision and embed robust supervision practice as opposed to those which overtly or inadvertently devalue and deprioritise supervision. We detect that the importance of a healthy pro-supervision culture is linked with the value managers and lead clinicians attribute to regular supervision opportunities and its pivotal relationship with high quality clinical practice. The relationship between supervision, a valued workforce and public safety appears to be appreciated by some leaders, however research which illustrates this connection would clearly strengthen the case for investment in supervision across healthcare. The link between the professional and financial value of supervision is seldom discussed. There is a sense from authors' accounts that there is a clear return on investment in supervision at personal, departmental, service and organisational levels which delivers both professional and public benefit. Furthermore, there is a case for joining the dots more clearly between protecting time for supervision and the impact on high level metrics like recruitment and retention, productivity, patient safety and health inequalities.

Exploring alternative approaches to supervision

We have been struck by the ways in which contributors have shown us an understanding of the breadth of professional supervision practice and the value of moving away from taken-for-granted and established ways of accessing professional supervision. There are examples which make the case for a mix of professional supervision approaches describing how these can serve the practitioner. These include group supervision, peer group supervision, cross-profession supervision, external supervision, supervision *in* and *on* practice and supervision *of* supervision. Authors show the scope and value of being experimental and highlight the need to regularly review supervision arrangements and ensure these are constantly aligned with the practitioner's needs.

Matching supervisory practice to the needs of the supervisees

A powerful aspect of this collection is that it demonstrates how each practitioner is a multidimensional individual and, as such, each supervisory relationship needs to be a collaborative learning process for both supervisee and supervisor. The accounts included demonstrate that supervisors do not need to be all-knowing and skilful in every dimension of supervision. Of greater importance is the ability to be self-aware, reflective, committed to open dialogue with each supervisee and to value ongoing self-development as a supervisee and supervisor. Core to this is a willingness to stand in another's shoes, to see practice and experiences from a different standpoint and to strive to ensure that supervision is both socially and culturally accessible and inclusive. Supervision is typically construed as a space to reflect on what the supervisee is finding difficult. However, the accounts in this book strongly promote the value of moving beyond deficits and problems to finding a space in supervision to identify and celebrate what is going well. This is possible when supervisors create conditions of trust and equity. As role models, such supervisors are willing to share gaps in their own knowledge and understanding and embrace the insights and learning they gain through supervisory relationships.

No one size fits all in supervision. The chapters demonstrate the need to carefully negotiate what will meet each supervisee's supervision needs at different points in time. This includes the importance of being aware of social and cultural impacts on supervision practice and the structures of power, privilege and oppression. Many authors highlight the need for different types and approaches to supervision at certain points including pre-registration, at different career stages and transitions. People want and need to access different structures at different stages, broadening out their options over the course of their career.

Ensuring practitioners are well equipped for practice

From chapter to chapter we notice differing supervision foci. Some authors share their experiences in highly technical contexts where there is the potential for the knowledge and skills of the speech and language therapist to overlap with other registered professionals in the interprofessional team. From mental health to critical care, these contexts involve navigating indistinct boundaries which include practitioner capability, professional scopes of practice, professional identities and practitioner wellbeing. Each element may require supervision and each aspect of supervision will be interrelated. Other authors demonstrate how supervision for technical knowledge and skills can support a practitioner's confidence in practice, their sense of professional self/identity and ultimately their personal and professional wellbeing. Similarly, supervision which provides a protected and trusted space to share and explore professional uncertainty can support the restoration of confidence in a practitioner's technical knowledge and skills. What is apparent from the chapters in this book is that there is a need in supervision to consider the practitioner as a whole human, practising and experiencing an extraordinary plethora of technical and knowledge-informed interactions in combination with intensely human encounters. As two of our contributors note, "the expectation that we can be immersed in suffering and loss daily and not be touched by it is as unrealistic as expecting to be able to walk through water without getting wet" (Remen, 1996, 96).

It is our core belief that supervision has a fundamental role in sustaining you through the intensity and demands of everyday practice. We hope this book broadens your outlook and offers alternative ways in which you can take new ideas forward into your own supervision, practice and organisational culture.

Reference

Remen, R. N. (1996). *Kitchen Table Wisdom: Stories That Heal*. Riverhead Books.

Climbing Out of the Window

Finding Supervision

Zein Pereira

When, as a lead speech and language therapy (SLT) clinician, I started asking questions about non-managerial supervision for lead clinicians and then requested non-managerial supervision for myself, it raised a few eyebrows.

The established culture in the organisation within which I had worked for 19 years, viewed regular non-managerial, or what is now called professional supervision (RCSLT, 2017) as primarily about competence and capability, and not appropriate for an experienced clinician, like me. My knowledge of professional supervision was formulated and embedded through this culture, and I had not come across alternative points of view through my initial training, any courses attended or interacting with allied health colleagues. My perspective was that professional supervision, at its core, was for less experienced staff and the content centred on clinical knowledge, clarifying points of procedure or policy and task focussed problem solving, not self-care. If there was a development need, this was dealt with through the (annual) appraisal-style proforma which directed the conversation to identifying targets, possibly including a course, a shadowing opportunity, or a journal article to read. Skills that a lead clinician should already possess, and therefore did not need professional supervision, surely?

This chapter reflects how I glimpsed what else supervision could be and made the decision to step outside of this culture to prioritise self-care and learn more. The effects of this decision continue to reverberate today.

I loved my job as a lead paediatric speech and language therapist, working for the National Health Service (NHS) in a specialist educational context. Common to all my SLT roles, the job had a breadth and depth of both mental and emotional demands. I had managerial and lead clinician responsibilities. I worked with motivated, focussed colleagues who faced the

DOI: 10.4324/9781003301141-1

1

complexities and pressures of their roles with inspiring volumes of energy, skill, creativity, and determination.

The paediatric SLT department allocated a lead clinician for each service area. As a lead clinician, I was managing my own caseload, with oversight for other caseloads, training others, advising, troubleshooting, developing service policy and procedures, and supporting a small team of therapists that I line managed. I also followed up on clinically complex second opinions and safeguarding concerns. As lead clinicians, supporting others was a core part of each of our roles. Support, enable, facilitate, advise, devise, co-ordinate, and develop others. . . . It was all there in the job description.

When additional challenges arose, such as gaps in staffing, there was usually a defined endpoint in sight. Typically, as the lead, I reviewed the needs of the individuals on the designated caseloads and made a plan that would see us through this short-term bump in the road. However, during a particularly challenging year when gaps in staffing started to overlap and remain uncovered, other challenges and demands started to stack up and embed themselves as a new normal in my week and the next week and the next week. The weeks turned into months, and without a clear endpoint, my resources began to deplete.

I had worked in this same organisation for nearly two decades. Large caseloads and short staffing were not a new phenomenon. I was working in an area of clinical practice where the children with severe to profound communication needs required intensive direct therapy. Our school-based caseloads were considered small to accommodate this. The small caseloads meant that we already had more clinical time per child than therapists in other clinical areas across the department. This in turn meant that we were not necessarily viewed as a priority for staffing cover. I knew that other lead clinicians were also stretched and trying their best to deliver a quality service, in the context of short staffing. Through our lead clinician meetings and informal liaison, we talked about ways of dealing with gaps in staffing, prioritising, and re-prioritising and then formulating priority plans. We did not really talk very much about how we felt about delivering those plans. Whatever the pressures, I thought it was my job to just get on with it. I thought the other lead clinicians were trying to just get on with it too. When I liaised with my managers about my prioritisation plans, they were extremely stretched too but also seemed to me to be getting on with it. So that is what I tried to do, *get on with it*. I wrote lists. I researched time management techniques. I delegated, though this inevitably created further work in terms of reassessment and monitoring. I sent out updates to parents about the staffing situation. I arrived early and left late. That was when it started to spill over into my home life. I worked at weekends. I went home late each weekday and within minutes of arriving home, I would start on a loop, talking about how I was feeling about work. Obviously, I could not talk about anything clinical or confidential, but the now chronic worry, frustration, and fatigue was at times, overwhelming. It affected my sleep patterns and I felt tired all the time. Recently when I asked my partner about what that time was like for her, she reminded me of when she tried to help me contain the stress, asking if she could set the kitchen timer to 30 minutes, my time limit for talking about work when I got home. This did provide some relief and helped me to stop filling every evening with talk about work, but it was not enough.

In 2008, nine years before the Royal College of Speech and Language Therapists (RCSLT) information on supervision was published in 2017, I read an article about supervision in *Speech and Language Therapy in Practice*, that opened my awareness of regular professional supervision being for everyone. The article defined supervision as somewhere to talk about one's work, whatever one's level of experience. This is what I needed. Somewhere supportive and enabling, somewhere I could leave feeling better than when I arrived. As a lead clinician, with the caseload, advisory and staffing responsibilities that the role entailed, it felt important to invest the time to talk about my work with someone who was not my manager.

So, in one lead clinician meeting, I asked about regular professional supervision for lead clinicians. It could be very useful I said, to be able to talk about our work with one another, to learn from and support one another. There was an audible pause then one of the managers said: 'I would not have expected you to need regular supervision, you always seem so competent'. And there it was, supervision was about competence or perhaps incompetence. In the moments following that remark, I felt so isolated and *incompetent*. To *need* supervision as an experienced practitioner was to have your competence questioned. The manager was not being deliberately negative or dismissive. She was merely reflecting the prevailing culture, where supervision was closely bound up with levels of experience and competence. Doubts flooded into my head. Who, in this group, needed supervision to process and reflect on the demands and challenges of their work? Were we all stressed and over stretched? Was I up to the job? No-one else was asking for professional supervision. Who had the time to fit in offering supervision to an experienced practitioner? I swallowed my discomfort and persisted, wondering out loud about the professional supervision needs of the whole service. How would it be if we could develop a supervision policy to encompass *everyone*, because we were all working in pressurised and at times, challenging circumstances and within that, fielding multiple demands, so we needed somewhere to take our thoughts, reflections, and (dare I say it) emotions. Somewhere to talk about our work to ensure we were offering the very best service possible. This was received with more recognition and initiated an intent to develop service supervision skills, structures, and guidelines. We spoke about it at the next paediatric staff meeting and there was a mixed response. Many staff looked weary as this was yet another demand on their time. Some said they did not need to be supervised. I sensed a prickly suspicion in the air. Was this about surveillance? They felt they could reflect on their own. Surely, being reflective was part of everyday practice and they certainly did not need yet another meeting to swallow up their precious time. Nonetheless, and to my relief, the manager stepped in, and we began the process of expanding our awareness and developing professional supervision for everyone in the SLT paediatric service.

As part of the process for developing staff guidelines, it was agreed that I contact one of the authors of the article I had read, to explore options for training for the whole department. We needed to be able to make the most of the supervision we were going to be attending and delivering on a regular basis. If we were going to schedule time away from clinical commitments, we needed to know what to do with it, so it was of genuine value. A series of conversations began that progressed into the planning of a training event for all of us. However, at the last moment, the service managers changed their minds and the plans for training were shelved in favour of preparing a guidance document to present at a staff meeting. I was so disappointed to lose the opportunity to train and build awareness of professional supervision together. Although I was asked to be involved in contributing to the supervision document, I felt that the presentation of a document within a staff meeting agenda was probably not going to change our fundamental supervision culture nor equip us with the awareness and skills we needed to learn. In due course, the draft document was presented at a staff meeting and a new regime of pairing people up for peer supervision was initiated. However, the arrangements for how lead clinicians might access regular supervision remained unclear. I broached the idea of swapping peer supervision in specialisms across other health providers, as it could be an issue for other lead clinicians across the NHS. However, the head of service made it clear that she was not comfortable with allowing external supervision as it was akin to washing our dirty laundry in public. At this point I wonder if I could have sought support from other professionals in this or other NHS departments. However, at that time, I could not see these alternatives and so remained participating in supporting others' supervision but without professional supervision for myself.

In many ways it was the perfect storm. One Friday morning, I realised that I had sat in my car in the work carpark, at 7.30 a.m. every day that week for a few moments longer each time. To even enter the building, I had needed to gather myself, to regroup and summon the mental energy to begin my working day. It creeps up on you, burnout, and I was on the edge of it, with rapidly depleting mental and physical resources. I remember being told as a child, when life closes a door, a window opens. I really did feel like I was standing in front of a closed door, and I could not stay standing there, something needed to change. Chronic staffing gaps remained uncovered, and a regular way of helping me to proactively manage my stress levels through skilled work-based supervision was now unlikely to materialise. I was exhausted and beginning to worry about my health. I decided that if I could find the metaphorical open window, I needed to climb out of it, and get some help! I had had several conversations with an independent supervisor regarding the supervision training and I felt that it was worth following this up myself and investing in my own health. So, dirty laundry or no dirty laundry, I decided to book an independent supervision session with this supervisor, external to my work context. With the benefit of hindsight, I could have also sought support from Occupational Health or via my General Practitioner, but at the time, I did not think it had gone that far.

In July 2009 I booked an annual leave day and boarded a train to London. The act of getting on a train to travel to a neutral space to try to feel better about my job felt like a very big step to take. We met in an open but private space in the Royal Festival Hall and settled in some comfortable chairs at a table. I felt anxious and I had no idea what to expect. The supervisor proceeded gently and with curiosity as we began to get to know each other so the session began with describing my supervision history. I tried to set the scene, and this included explaining my professional supervision history after 19 years of practice. This did not take long! I received supervision as a newly qualified practitioner, and in the last year I had a few sessions with my manager to talk about a very specific and particularly complex work-related situation. I had joined peer support groups, I had managerial meetings, I accessed informal support and had regular time by the kettle with colleagues, but as an experienced practitioner, I had not had professional supervision, ever.

That first session of independent supervision was a bit of a blur, but I do remember that after just one session, I felt better. I started to understand that professional supervision is about learning and critically for me, also about self-care. I felt relieved, lighter, and listened to. At the end of the session, I felt that I could return to work with hope and a sense of renewal which, at that stage, was less about specific strategies or actions and more about how I felt.

I booked another independent supervision session and felt certain that I wanted my discovery of supervision to continue. Our next session was on the phone as we were geographically far apart. It is arguably more difficult to set up a space that feels safe, on the phone, without the ongoing face-to-face interaction. However, the space did feel safe and non-judgemental, and this inspired a trust which underpinned all our sessions. Self-care had been the original driver to seek external professional supervision, and this continued as an intrinsic theme in the supervision process. I continued to book regular sessions and as well as feeling more supported, I was learning a lot about supervision and about myself as a therapist.

One immediate puzzle was what I should bring to my professional supervision sessions. In the current information on supervision (RCSLT, 2017), there is a list of themes and topics that one can bring to professional supervision, but at the time, with my limited experience of supervision, it felt like an unspoken rule to stick as closely as possible to clinical issues and avoid anything *personal*. However, as a lead clinician, I wanted to engage critically with all the issues in my work context and the supervisor made it clear that I could bring whatever I needed to, it could be a clinical case, a complex dilemma, discomfort in relation to a work dynamic or a single worry. This fact alone, feeling free to bring anything related to my work, including how I felt, created a sense of calm and relief. I no longer felt isolated, even though the supervisor did not share the same clinical speciality. Whatever I brought, that is where we began and we stayed with it until something shifted, which could take five minutes, twenty minutes, or the whole hour. We focused in to take it apart, get inside it and understand it. We broadened out to consider the context from different angles with the goal of deepening our understanding of what I was grappling with. The supervisor facilitated the session in ways that I did not expect, such as naming and clarifying everything in a very explicit way, encouraging curiosity, and supporting me to examine my values. I was struck by how the supervisor carefully checked and challenged what I meant by the everyday words I used, assuming nothing and enabling me to take a step back and critically examine the familiar (Shohet, 2011).

Such explicit examination was something I might have done when explaining a rationale, procedure, or approach to a student. The process in clinical education where one tries to make one's knowledge and ways of doing something, visible, both in theoretical and practical terms. As an experienced clinician, to unpack and name what had become tacit through repetition and do this for my own benefit, was a gamechanger for me. This process of identifying and revisiting the layers and angles within an approach, clarifying and reclarifying what I meant, attending to what happened and making it more and more explicit, felt grounding and enabling. It helped me to notice unnamed assumptions and habits, however small. This explicitness helped me to reflect more critically, develop my curiosity, notice more about myself, and learn fresh, enhanced perspectives, for example how my definition of being 'hard working' might affect my approach to managing a backlog. I could have attempted this on my own, but I think this would have been self-limiting. My own reflections may not have been as detailed, may have led to me rationalising my existing practice and only getting my own perspective back (McCormick, in Stokes & McCormick, 2015).

As an experienced clinician, discovering a renewed curiosity through the process of supervision, noticing, and observing my practice and myself in my practice in the middle of an extremely stressful period, felt transformative. Curiosity felt energising not exhausting and enabled me to deal with myself and any areas that felt stuck with a gentle, determined, persistence. Supervision helped me to see how I could turn curiosity into action in terms of setting small personal experiments, for example scheduling my diary differently, allowing more time for a dialogue with families and colleagues, and negotiating with others to enable further collaboration around service delivery. Added to that were small but important common-sense changes for my self-care, such as drinking enough water, eating lunch away from my desk and going home on time, all aspects that had become neglected through stress. I believe that renewing my curiosity about myself in work, was key in helping me to manage stress and dragged me back from the brink of burnout.

Another surprise as I worked with the supervisor was how central my values were and how they figured in what I brought to the session. Egan (cited by McCormick, in Stokes & McCormick, 2015) describes values, not as ideals but as a set of practical criteria that we use to support our decision making and drive our behaviour. This became apparent with a supervisor who could help me consider the complexities of my work and my responses through explicitly exploring my values and attitudes. This enabled me to see the lens that I looked through as the therapist that I was in my work context, and perhaps the therapist I could become.

I think I assumed that as an experienced speech and language therapist, I could just use my existing skills, but I realised there was a lot to learn so I invested in attending supervision training. This helped me to develop my awareness and understanding of the processes involved, and what good supervision looks like. Learning about a developmental model of supervision enabled me to examine my inexperience as a supervisee in relation to stages of development from novice through to fully mature supervisee (Simpson & Sparkes, 2008). Incidentally, this feels like an infinite work in progress! The more advanced supervision training deepened my understanding and allowed me the space to practise the component skills as both a supervisee and a supervisor. Certainly, the modelling and insights gained by listening to and observing colleagues, was invaluable in clarifying alternatives to the problem-solving, advisory type of approach that I had previously been used to. I continued to invest in training and as I would in my clinical work, I also invested in broader learning opportunities that could usefully enrich my knowledge and skills. For example, courses in Personal Construct Psychology and coaching.

Three years after that first independent supervision session, I resigned from my lead clinician role in the NHS. The uncovered staffing shortages continued, and services were about to be reorganised around this to become much more consultative and delegated, with less joint working than I was comfortable with. At that point, regular professional supervision for lead clinicians had still not become established as the norm. I cited this as one of my reasons for leaving. Ultimately, I needed to respect my professional values and prioritise my self-care to continue to work as a speech and language therapist. Without the independent supervision I accessed during those three years, I feel certain that I would have left the profession, burnt out. Ironically, good quality professional supervision gave me the confidence to respect my professional values and prioritise my self-care, which ultimately led to my resignation.

I now work independently as a clinician and a supervisor. The increased use of online platforms has enabled me to work with a range of people from different areas, in addition to in-person sessions. The ongoing development of my knowledge and skills and the expansion of my work as a supervisor, give me joy! Supervision is as essential to my practice and my wellbeing as ever. I continue to regularly access professional supervision both one to one and in a group. My one-to-one supervision is a combination of alternate self-funded sessions and peer supervision with an independent colleague. The cumulative and ongoing effect of such investment, and learning opportunities that offer depth and breadth, has influenced my work across the board. It affects how I reflect and collaborate with families and professionals. For example, I have noticed that I listen for longer, ask different questions, assume less, and check my understanding more explicitly. I certainly allow more time for the conversations and negotiations needed to move forward and make progress.

Concluding thoughts

I recently asked my partner what she thought of that time before I climbed out of the metaphorical window and how it is for her now, compared to then. She said, there is no comparison. She said that when I climbed out of that window, I took ownership and then made choices that took me out of a system that was not listening. She said that changing my work context created new possibilities that positively affected my well-being. She said that there is no need to set the kitchen timer now, and best of all, it is good to see me as happy in work, as in life.

This feels like an important note to close with. I strongly feel that as health professionals, whatever our clinical backgrounds and wherever we are geographically, we need somewhere to talk about our work. However, supervision is as much about self-care and wellbeing as anything else. We need somewhere to reflect, not just on our work, but on ourselves in our work.

This includes how we feel, because that fundamentally affects not just our wellbeing, but how we work with others.

References

Shohet, R. (ed) (2011). *Supervision as Transformation, A Passion for Learning*. London: Jessica Kingsley.

Simpson, S. & Sparkes, C. (2008) Are you getting enough? – (1) Supervision in context. *Speech and Language Therapy in Practice.*

Stokes, J. & McCormick, M. (eds) (2015). *Speech and Language Therapy and Professional Identity: Challenging Received Wisdom*. London: J & R Press Ltd.

Royal College of Speech & Language Therapists (RCSLT) (2017). Information on Supervision.

2

The Role of Supervision in Supporting and Empowering Patient Voice and Choice

Scott Ballard-Ridley

My experiences as a clinician, patient and health improvement trainer have shaped my views about supervision. I qualified as a physiotherapist in 2006 and was first introduced to the concept of supervision during my training. Shortly after qualifying I suffered a major stroke which left me with a chronic condition that I would need to manage for the rest of my life. I returned to work in health services, initially as an administrator for a community therapy team. I am now employed in a social enterprise as a healthcare improvement trainer and work with healthcare professionals and UK National Health Service (NHS) policy forums with a focus on how to work collaboratively with patients to achieve better outcomes. Supervision continues to play a huge role in my life personally and professionally.

I do not think most members of the public know much about supervision or that the healthcare professionals they see have a professional responsibility to seek regular supervision. I cannot help but feel that if this were known more widely, the public would be professional supervision's strongest advocates. In this chapter, I make my case for the value of supervision for health professionals using personal insights and illustrations.

The influence of supervision experiences in shaping interactions with patients

As a healthcare improvement trainer, I work with clinicians to support ways of working more collaboratively with patients to encourage greater self-management. A central part of the training is to encourage clinicians to

DOI: 10.4324/9781003301141-2

work in a person-focused way. The sessions are co-facilitated by somebody with learned experience and somebody with lived experience, like me. My role is to bring the self-management theories and concepts we introduce to life through my own lived experience. I notice that clinicians often seem to find the lived experience aspect of the training uncomfortable. I sense this happens because the clinicians begin to realise that they are not working in the most patient-focused way, although they may previously have thought they were. I also observe that the clinicians who make the most progress and maybe even the biggest changes to their practice, both during the training and after, are the ones who tell us they have robust support mechanisms in place, through for example, supervision.

Many of the clinicians who attend the training are allied health professionals (AHPs). In the UK, AHPs are required to engage in regular, effective supervision to ensure they work within their scope of practice (HCPC, 2023). In my view, supervision is effective when it provides a safe space to talk about practice. I observe that clinicians who have this safe space to explore new ideas and reflect on their practice in a non-judgemental way are far more likely to model this way of working with their patients. A further feature of effective supervision is that it focuses on the supervisee, seeing the person in the clinician (Rothwell et al., 2021). In my view, clinicians who experience supervision which is clinician-focused and encourages professional growth will apply this approach in their clinical practice too. Something that seems important to me is differentiating managerial and professional supervision. I notice that supervisors are not always able to do this. I accept that there needs to be a balance, but I am concerned that it will be difficult for a supervisee to think about their own practice, hopes and fears if their supervisor focuses on productivity and caseload targets.

I think I can spot the clinicians who take their learning in supervision forward into their practice. Their positive supervision interactions seamlessly start to influence their interactions with patients. An important indicator of this influence is the way in which I hear clinicians talk about their patients. Clinicians whose language for activities like supervision is the same as the language they use for patient and public-facing activities really stand out. It cheers me when, instead of talking about a patient in terms of a condition and impairments, 'the 67-year-old stroke in bed 9', I hear things like 'Bob, the 67-year-old man who likes gardening and is keen to get back to this following his stroke'. In this description, I hear a willingness on the part of the clinician to acknowledge and talk about hopes and fears with patients; an important aspect of encouraging self-management. It seems to me that if a supervisor models compassion in supervision, the supervisee is more likely to be a compassionate clinician. If supervisors apply a 'what matters to my supervisee' approach, then their supervisees are more likely to apply a 'what matters to my patient' approach. If a supervisor is willing to talk with a supervisee about challenges, hopes and fears then the clinician may feel more prepared to do the same with patients. Through supervision, the language of compassion and person-focus can become both normalised, socialised and embedded in practice.

Collaboration not combat

All too often in healthcare I feel the power dynamic is tipped in favour of the clinician. For example, not long after I left hospital following my stroke, I worked with a local senior neurological physiotherapist for help with my mobility. Please note that I describe this as 'working with a physiotherapist' not 'having physiotherapy' as this sort of relationship is often described. Through a friend, I was offered a consultation with another senior physiotherapist in a different area of the country. My stroke changed my life dramatically and I was keen to hear from anyone who might have helpful guidance for me about my mobility, so I took up the opportunity. I was offered the consultation rather than seeking it, but it could nonetheless be described as getting a second opinion. I have heard clinicians talk about second opinions in a dismissive way, perhaps feeling a second opinion is an indication that the patient does not trust them. My view is that we all have a right to make decisions about our healthcare, including whether we choose to seek other points of view. In the spirit of working *with* the local neurophysiotherapist, I shared some thoughts I had gained from my additional consultation. The local clinician was furious and indicated I had gone behind her back. My motivation had not been to challenge practice, but to exercise my right to have control over decisions about my own wellbeing.

I have reflected on this interaction and on the way I use my own professional supervision to explore alternative perspectives about, for example, tricky professional relationships. This approach in supervision has helped me to see things from another person's perspective and work out ways to improve relationships, such as presenting things in a way that the other person might better understand. Looking back, I wonder what role supervision might have had in supporting the local physiotherapist to have an alternative conversation with me. Instead of being angry with me, might the physiotherapist have talked through her feelings with her supervisor in the first instance? If her supervision was safe and effective, might the supervisor have supported her to 'stand in my shoes'? Might this have encouraged her to explore my motivations to seek a second opinion and look collaboratively at the ideas I returned with to help identify how these, in combination with her own, could help me manage my mobility? Might we have had a conversation about my mobility hopes and fears? I like to think that a senior clinician feeling perhaps that their professional opinion had been questioned by the patient would take this to supervision for further reflection rather than take their frustration out on their patient, who is perfectly within their rights to seek a second opinion. This is not just my opinion. At the time of writing, the UK Patient Safety Commissioner (PSC, no date) are consulting on the introduction of Martha's Rule which will ensure patients', families' and carers' views and voices are central to their care. Effective supervisors recognise they learn from and with their supervisees and modelling this idea of two experts in the room is vital for collaborative clinician-patient interactions.

Patients want to know their clinicians are being looked after

So far, I have focused on the ways in which supervision can influence interactions with patients, but there is also an important clinician wellbeing part of supervision. There are many examples, especially throughout the Covid-19 pandemic, of how the public holds our healthcare workforce in high regard. People want to know healthcare workers are being looked after. According to the Health Foundation (2022), 'people's top priorities for the National Health Service (NHS) include addressing the workload pressures on NHS staff, increasing the number of staff in the NHS and improving waits for routine services'. I suggest that one of the most effective ways for an employer to ensure that staff's emotional and mental wellbeing needs are being met is through effective professional supervision, which, as I have described, provides a safe space for discussion and the opportunity to explore new possibilities. A review of research by Martin et al. (2021) indicates health professionals also see professional supervision as an important factor in reducing stress and burnout, reducing the numbers of staff leaving the healthcare workforce and improving the work environment. When, from my patient perspective, I hear and read that there is a record shortfall in the global healthcare workforce (World Health Organisation, 2023) investing in effective supervision seems like an important way for healthcare employers to show that the workforce is valued.

In my work as a healthcare improvement trainer, one of the goals of our sessions is to provide teams with an hour a week to focus on themselves and their team. Most teams say that this protected time for reflection and planning is one of the things they value most about the training as they do not usually make time for this in their daily work. Time and space for reflection is a key aspect of effective supervision and supporting best practice. If the public were aware of this, they would, in an act of role reversal, be 'prescribing' supervision for their healthcare professionals.

Research indicates that patients are becoming more complex, requiring more interventions and the workforce is being expected to manage this with much less resource (The King's Fund, 2021). Many of the clinicians I work with as an improvement trainer describe taking on board the fears and concerns of the patients they work with and making them their own. Just after my stroke when I was an inpatient, I had some considerable fears about what the future held for me. I did not feel that I could share these fears with my close friends and family at the time because I felt that they already had so much on their plate, so I shared them with my therapy team and immediately had a sense of relief. This sharing of hopes and fears was vital for me being able to progress with my therapy. Had I held onto these concerns I believe my outcomes would have suffered. I recognise now how important it would be for those clinicians to have an appropriate outlet to share the emotional load of their work through effective supervision. If I found myself in a similar position now and knew that my clinicians did not have effective supervision in place, I would worry that the clinicians were not sufficiently supported to be able to take on board the sensitive information I wanted to share and I would hold back from sharing it.

Concluding thoughts

Looking back on nearly a decade of work as a healthcare improvement trainer, I notice that the clinicians and teams that have been best placed and most willing to adopt positive change for themselves and their patients are the ones who describe having a strong support culture. I have also observed that the teams with a robust supervision structure throughout the team, from the administrator to the team lead, have the best patient feedback data and the highest levels of staff satisfaction. These teams are the ones that differentiate between managerial supervision and professional supervision. These teams are few and far between, but when you come across them you really know. These teams, and by extension their clinicians, are the ones that are all rowing in the same direction, are not afraid to think outside of the box to meet the needs of the patient but maybe, most importantly of all, have the highest number of people with a smile on their face. Finally, I often talk with clinicians about what good outcomes look like. Sometimes I have heard clinicians say that it is when a patient says, 'I couldn't have done this without you'. While this can make the clinician feel valued, it implies that the patient's success is uniquely down to the clinician. A true marker of success is to hear: 'Thank you for empowering me to be successful'. I suggest that the same probably applies when evaluating whether supervision has been effective.

References

HCPC (2023) *Standards of Proficiency for Practice*. Available online at: www.hcpc-uk.org/standards/standards-of-proficiency/ [Last accessed: 29/11/2023].

Health Foundation (2022) *Public Perceptions of the NHS and Social Care: Performance, Policy and Expectations*. Available online at: www.health.org.uk/publications/long-reads/public-perceptions-performance-policy-and-expectations [Last accessed: 17.08.23].

The King's Fund (2021) *Addressing Complex Needs in the Community: A GP Trainee's Perspective*. Available online at: www.kingsfund.org.uk/blog/2021/11/addressing-complex-needs-community-gp-trainees-perspective [Last accessed: 17.08.23].

Martin P, Lizarondo L, Kumar S, Snowdon D. (2021) Impact of clinical supervision on healthcare organisational outcomes: A mixed methods systematic review. *PLoS One*, 16(11): e0260156. doi:10.1371/journal.pone.0260156.

PSC (no date) Patient Safety Commissioner. Available online at: https://www.patientsafetycommissioner.org.uk/ [Last accessed: 29.11.23].

Rothwell C., Kehoe A., Farook S.F. & Illing J. (2021) Enablers and barriers to effective clinical supervision in the workplace: A rapid evidence review. *BMJ Open*, 11(9): e052929. doi:10.1136/bmjopen-2021-052929.

World Health Organisation (2023) *Health Topics: Health Workforce*. Available online at: www.who.int/health-topics/health-workforce#tab=tab_1 [Last accessed: 17.08.23].

3 | Supervision in Pre-registration Speech and Language Therapy Education

Melanie Packer

I started working in the speech and language therapy (SLT) profession in 2001. I remember my first interview at that time, for a post as a speech and language therapy assistant. Who knew what my career trajectory would be like? I certainly had no idea that 20 years later I would be employed by a university that delivers pre-registration SLT courses. I looked different to the women that I worked alongside: Being a person of dual heritage background and a single mother left me feeling like an outsider. The women that I worked with were white and predominantly married or in a committed relationship. So, when I joined the team, fears of not belonging were amplified by my difference. Despite my apprehension, I was made welcome by a team, for the first time, I was beginning to find my professional tribe. Eventually I returned to university to train as a speech and language therapist.

From the moment that I took on the role as an assistant, fears of falling short of both cultural and professional requirements, sparked my curiosity. Instinctively I began to reflect and seek advice through shared reflections and discussion. What I then feared as my weaknesses, or perceived shortcomings, I perceive now as the catalyst for my career and the therapist and lecturer that I am today. However, in the early stages of my career, including placements, I thought that I had to present myself as the finished product. I did not appreciate that the best way to learn was to accept myself as a learner.

Q. Did I receive supervision whilst on placement?
A. Sometimes
Q. Did I always know that it was 'supervision'?
A. Probably not.

DOI: 10.4324/9781003301141-3

Q. Did my practice educators cue me in, 'I'm about to give you feedback' or plan or encourage me to seek specific times for supervision?

A. Not that I recall.

Q. Did *all* my practice educators provide good quality supervision?

A. An interesting question.

As a newly qualified therapist, competencies were signed off within the expected time frame, but I am not sure that I felt reassured that I was making progress. I left my first band 6 role much earlier than expected. Regular supervision might have enabled me to continue in that role. Subsequent employment changed my understanding of professional supervision, as it was the first post where professional supervision was firmly scheduled within my diary. It was a normal part of practice: expected and protected, so much so, that when I changed teams or employer, if it were not offered, I would seek it. I came to supervision just in time. Without it, I know that I would not have stayed in the profession.

Embedding supervision into practice placements.

In this chapter, the term supervision and professional supervision are used interchangeably to refer to a learning relationship that enables ongoing development of knowledge and skills associated with clinical and professionals practice, as defined by RCSLT (2023b). It is distinct from managerial supervision which refers to 'line management supervision' (RCSLT, 2023b). It is worth noting that this distinction is not delineated within RCSLT's (2021b) guidance for practice-based learning. Whilst training, the guidance states that SLT students' 100 out of 150 placement sessions should be supervised by a qualified speech and language therapist (RCSLT, 2021b).

However, what constitutes direct supervision within those 100 sessions is appears to be open to interpretation by practice educators and Higher Education Institutes (HEIs). Furthermore, the extent to which direct supervision is defined as managerial, professional supervision, or simply acknowledgment that the student is observed, is perhaps reliant upon the individual therapist/ practice educator and their interpretation of what is expected for that placement. Nor is direct supervision defined by the practice educators' proximity to the student (RCSLT 2021b). Increasingly, since the onset of COVID-19, there has been recognition that direct supervision could take place virtually. Whilst a student may be located in environments such as a school, the practice educator (the qualified speech and language therapist) may supervise remotely. Where this is the case reflection upon for the student's stage of development, the nature of the environment and client group, along with the student's readiness to be supported in this way must be given serious consideration.

From a student perspective, variation in interpretation of what is direct supervision can lead to ambiguity within the student-practice educator relationship and the expectations of each party. They may also notice differences in their experience compared to their peers. Arguably student direct supervision should be aligned with expectations of professional supervision for any qualified speech and language therapist, as defined by RCSLT Guidance: 'What is Supervision?' (RCSLT, 2021a). However, an implicit power relationship frequently exists between the student and educators, as frequently the student's educator is also the practice assessor and for some students and educators this can be problematic. How does an assessor detach themselves, so they can support in a non-judgmental manner and then determine whether a student has indeed passed their placement? Students tell me that they are often painfully aware that the paradoxical nature of the practice assessor-educator role can have a negative impact, making it difficult for both educator and student to establish trust as a good foundation for learning and supervision.

Thankfully, there are many practice educators and students who manage to establish positive relationships and a suitable balance between the assessor-educator role. Spencer and Healey (2022) provide a useful definition that could be used to help us understand what is meant by direct supervision, recognising that like any form of communication, supervision is a two-way process and therefore successful supervision is dependent upon both students and educators being active participants in the process of supervision. Whilst students need to be proactive in preparing for and engaging in supervision, as well as completing subsequent actions. The educator's role is to offer guidance, challenge and support, identifying student's current level of skill and therefore appropriate activity for the student moving forward (Spencer & Healey, 2022).

As an educator, I advocate for supervision to be valued as an integral part of SLT practice education and clinical placements. It is necessary for the profession to ensure that SLT students receive good quality supervision from the very beginning of their professional careers (RCSLT, 2021a). RCSLT

(2023b) provides clear guidelines on the supervision that newly qualified therapists should receive and makes a distinction between managerial and professional supervision. However, the newly qualified practitioner's experience does not start at the point of qualification. Professional identity formation commences in the first year of study (Tucker, 2023). The therapist's career starts in training.

It is widely accepted that professional supervision and associated training is crucial to professional development (RCSLT, 2023b; HCPC, 2022a; HCPC, 2022b; Harding, 2019; Stokes, 2015; Geller, 2015). There is also recognition that adequate clinical supervision is an area which has been neglected in SLT training (Stokes, 2015). This chapter focuses upon supervision whilst SLT students are on placement, though acknowledges that teaching on the subject of supervision and opportunities to practise has its place in the classroom also. A consistent approach to supervision is required for both student and qualified speech and language therapists. If best practice is to separate managerial and professional supervision for qualified speech and language therapists (RCSLT, 2023b; Snowdon et al., 2020), it is necessary for students also.

During placement debriefs students have commented on how practice placements provide ideal opportunities for students to both observe and experience supervision. Firstly, observing supervision on placement supports student appreciation of supervision as a professional requirement. Secondly, supervision also serves as a learning tool that supports the student's own professional development. In classroom teaching, students are routinely exposed to the premise that therapists use interpersonal skills to establish trust, understanding and connection with clients, carers, and work colleagues. They also benefit from understanding the barriers that can devalue the relationship that they seek to establish or sustain. Perhaps less explored is the possibility of uncertainty in practice (Harding, 2019). Do practice educators openly discuss the vulnerability that they may experience in practice and what the triggers for this may be? Without allowing for vulnerability the capacity for empathy is diminished (Brown, 2018). Similarly, students are faced repeatedly with new and challenging scenarios whilst engaging in clinical activity that inevitability brings into question their emerging practice. Explicit exploration of potential triggers through supervision is pertinent for placement. Allowing students to define and manage emotions and thoughts experienced through a process of discussion, without fear of being judged, is as important as exploring underpinning theoretical knowledge.

This is particularly useful for those students who perceive vulnerability and uncertainty as a weakness.

The profession requires 'compassionate leaders', as defined by West (2021). Speech and language therapists therefore have a responsibility to prepare a future workforce that is attuned to high levels of self-awareness, awareness of others, as well as the skills and processes that enable speech and language therapists to navigate challenging contexts, whilst sustaining best practice. Baxter (2004) refers to the 'hidden curriculum', as the development or socialisation of the professional self, asking practice educators to consider pre-registration students not as 'students' but as 'professionals in training'. Geller (2015) perceives 'professional use of self' as an integral part of SLT practice that requires nurturing and development through formal training and supervision.

Supervision on placement

Students fortunate enough to receive high quality supervision and witness speech and language therapists (practice educators) receiving supervision, such as group supervision, or observe impromptu professional support in the office, express how this serves as a process of normalisation, leading to its acceptance as a core part of practice. Students observe the skills that therapists utilise e.g., active listening, Socratic questioning, kindness. In addition, they witness the reasons for supervision and how the supervisee is received. Students have commented that being invited to group supervision sessions enabled the students to acknowledge that no one therapist will have all the answers, but group supervision could offer a range of alternative solutions.

It is recognised that all students should regularly receive supervision whilst on placement (RCSLT, 2021b). Spencer and Healey (2022) recommend a minimum of one hour per week, but they recognise that the supervision in healthcare may be more fragmented consisting of shorter episodes of supervision occurring across the week. Baxter (2004) makes explicit the tension between the students' opportunities to experience working independently in practice and opportunities for regular feedback. As discussed in section 2, the RCSLT (2021b) Practice Based Learning Guidance does not currently give specific recommendations regarding the frequency or nature of supervision for students. However, when planning for supervision for a forthcoming placement and determining how supervision will be offered, there are key factors that practice educators should consider:

- placement design,
- student's stage of professional development,
- clients' needs and safety,
- the clinical environment.

Supervision should enable the student to:

- Reflect and openly discuss the student's clinical involvement with specific clients.
- Demonstrate their understanding of theory in relation to the clients and their response to the clinical situations.
- Consider the client, carer, and the student's overall well-being.
- Evaluate performance during an activity or evaluate progress in relation to specific learning goals and continued professional development generally.

Observations lead me to conclude that students who do well on placement take ownership for their learning and identify next steps for their development; supervision provides an opportunity for thoughts and ideas to be worked through and reviewed in a subsequent meeting. It is the responsibility of the practice educator to facilitate this process. Based upon my experience of working as a speech and language therapist and lecturer, I recommend that specific roles and responsibilities are adopted. I recognise that there may be local variation. Figure 3.1 summarises these roles and responsibilities, followed by discussion in further detail in section 4.

Troubleshooting

Experience of working in a university has given me an overview of the practice-educator relationship. For some, establishing and maintaining a student-practice educator relationship can be straightforward. Where this is the case, the relationship is often effortless, with communication smooth and clear. Practice educators share feedback, notice that new learning is reflected upon and incorporated into the student's subsequent practice. The student makes expected progress.

	Student	Placement supervisor/ educator	HEI
Prior to placement/ start of placement	Attends University placement briefings. Identifies placement aims for the forthcoming placement. Identifies reflection tools to support discussion. Establishes methods for recording experiences and reflections once placement starts. Makes contact with practice educators prior to the start of placement.	Discusses students' expectations for supervision during placement. Negotiates a supervision plan with the student(s). Discusses with students the placement goals or aims that the student has identified for the placement and how these aims link to the placement assessment.	Supports the students to prepare for placement. Provides relevant practice educator training. Acts as a point of contact for practice educators.
During Placement	Prepares for supervision, identifying the key points for discussion in a forthcoming meeting (Spencer & Healey 2021). Books a physical or virtual space for meeting at an agreed time. Actively participates in reflection and evaluation of recent events and performance during supervision. Takes a positive approach to supervision and is open and honest in line with HCPC standards. Writes a meeting summary, including actions and shares the summary with her practice educator(s). Open to change / transformation.	Provides opportunities where the student is directedly observed, and appropriate, opportunities for independence. Protects time for supervision and feedback on the student's progress in relation to the learning goal.	Is at hand to provide supervision to students and practice educators.

Figure 3.1 Roles and responsibilities

Experience also tells me that educators and students do not always experience this smooth transaction within interactions. There are times when student-practice educator relationships are effortful. Miscommunication is more frequent, or communication infrequent and behaviours, whether the students' or the educators' are perceived as being undesirable. Students report and qualified speech and language therapists describe experiences that range from exceptionally positive to extremely negative, including reports of discrimination.

We may see natural synergies between ourselves and the students that we work with and at other times we may not. It is important to embrace the possibility that the presence or absence of connection between the student and practice educator is not necessarily an indication of a student's current knowledge, skills or potential. Working relationships are complex and student-educator relationships are no different. Our professional commitment to working collaboratively despite difference, addressing potential barriers to effective working should also be applied when educating the future workforce. Compassionately acknowledging the dynamic and unique relationship between educator and learner, as well as acknowledging uncertainty and mutual vulnerability, can go a long way to generating a more productive relationship. Personal experience of being a student on placement can be useful to draw upon, but it is essential that we also consider the contemporary context in which SLT students are now learning.

Student education takes up energy; physical, mental and emotional energy. An imbalance of energy can cause practice educators to question their own practice or doubt their observations of student behaviour(s). Arguably supervision for practice educators that focuses specifically on student support is a key part of providing high quality practice education. Practice educators require safe spaces to be 'held' or 'contained' in a way that enables the practice educator to explore pedagogical knowledge, as well as thoughts and feelings that may be triggered as a result of a placement experience (Geller, 2015). The type of support available to educators may vary depending on where they are based and the universities that they are affiliated to. Practice educators have a responsibility to liaise with the student's university if they have a concern or query. Speech and language therapists employed within a team can also reach out to peers, or a practice placement coordinator. The coordinator could be an allied health professional (AHP) placement manager, an AHP practice educator facilitator, or someone in the speech and language therapy department.

Finally, we must acknowledge that there are times when despite all efforts a placement can breakdown beyond repair. If this is the case, then it is essential that both the student and practice educators independently receive a placement debrief meeting that is provided by the university. Typically, the characteristics and functions of the debrief mirror supervision. Wherever possible, practice educators, students and university tutors work to prevent breakdown and aim to nurture supportive placements. Outlined below you will find ideas to help minimise potential barriers to a successful placement experience. The considerations below are based upon my professional experience. The approach taken may vary dependent on the partner universities and specific placement design.

Am I confident enough to be a supervisor?

Universities offer training and all practice educators should access training prior to having their first student on placement. Subsequent training can be accessed when required and it is recommended that all practice educators access training at least every three years (RCSLT, 2021b). If you are unsure and would like support, please contact the university that is local to you.

How can I manage student expectations and potential ambiguity regarding supervision on placement?

For some students this may be their first interaction in a professional health context. At the beginning of placement, it is important to:

- Ensure that roles and responsibilities are clearly explained.
- Confirm that the student(s) are clear about the topics that could be discussed in supervision and ask questions relating to the placement.
- Explain how you will give feedback. Wherever possible relate feedback back to learning outcomes or goals. This may go some way to ensure that students have insight into their ongoing development and helps maintain a certain level of objectivity to feedback received (Spencer and Healey, 2022).
- Ask the students to set the agenda for supervision meetings, record key items discussed including learning and actions point that have been generated as part of the supervision (Spencer and Healey, 2022).
- Ask the student to write a summary of the supervision meeting and provide you with a copy, so that there is a shared record and follow up actions can be reviewed at a later date (Spencer and Healey, 2022).

What if a student is not taking responsibility for their learning and supervision?

- Check that the student has a clear understanding of their responsibilities and those of the practice educators supporting them. Be clear that students are expected to be active in their own learning.
- If the student is not ready to lead in the process, model a proactive approach or provide a scaffold that enables the student(s) to take the lead over time.
- Check for potential barriers. e.g. Are there gaps in the student's understanding of the learning outcomes or goals for the placement? Equally there may be other factors such as health, travel, accommodation, and finance that may impede in the students' ability to engage in their own learning.
- Be explicit about how supervision links to continued professional development and one of RCSLT five core capabilities, 'Leadership and Lifelong Learning' and HCPC standards of proficiency.
- Students are painfully aware that practice educators are both teachers and assessors. Openly discuss this dual role and how it can be managed. For some students the 'fear of getting it wrong' can be overwhelming. Support students to develop a growth mindset, to regard learning as an iterative process that supervision aims to facilitate. Students must start as learners before they can be accomplished practitioners. Openly discuss how all clinicians learn from experience, which includes learning from mistakes. Give personal examples where possible.

What if I find it difficult to connect with a student(s)?

- Reflect on your interaction style and the expectations or demands that you may be explicitly or implicitly placing upon the student and yourself.
- Be realistic in your own abilities as a practice educator and seek advice or supervision.
- Be realistic for the student, focus on the stage of their development rather than expectations of what knowledge and skills they *should* be demonstrating.
- Work with the student(s) to identify the immediate next steps.
- Some students feel like they are being continually tested or judged. Reflect on the number of questions that you may be asking and

consider using a balance or questioning, pausing and comments. Are you valuing the student responses during supervision? Be mindful of how much our preferences influence our interpretation of a student's emerging skill.

- Ensure that both the learner's strengths as well as their learning needs are considered. Explore how they got confident in their existing skills. How can they draw on those learning experiences to address the less secure aspects of their practice?
- Identify individual or structural factors that may indirectly impact on the relationship and the supervision experience. Sensitively explore the student's lived experience now as a student or in previous employment or in education. Reflect on how these experiences impact on how they engage in supervision and or your perception of how they will engage.
- Acknowledge the socio-economic and political privileges we hold as qualified speech and language therapists. These may be inherited or acquired privileges. Identify conscious or unconscious biases that you hold and how these might impact upon the student–practice educator relationship and the outcome of placement.
- Reflect upon the personal or professional factors that can make it harder for you to meet the responsibilities of being a practice educator. Speak with your line manager or your team's practice coordinator if a reasonable adjustment is required, or if it is not the right time for you to support a student.

Am I fully supporting diversity in the future workforce?

Wider socio-economic and political factors and systemic structures may negatively impact on students experience on placement being considered. For example, 'The Broken Ladder' report (Gyimah et al., 2022) highlights the experiences of women of colour and their experience of entering the UK's workforce. Women of colour speak of negative assumptions regarding their capabilities, microaggressions in education and the workplace and the constant expenditure of mental energy required by women of colour to manage the context in which they work. This concept of additional mental and emotional energy expenditure impacting on academic life is acknowledged within the field of psychology as well as personal accounts (Steele, 1997; Kinouani, 2021; Grant, 2023; Packer, 2023). 'Experience of unbelonging'

(Gyimah et al., 2022), unfortunately starts in education. Women may feel forced to make changes to their physical appearance, to evade conversation topics or withhold aspects of their personality. The long-term consequence can be extreme; anxiety, depression, and departure from the profession that they seek to contribute to (Dabiri, 2019; Clarke et al., 2021; Gyimah et al., 2022; Packer, 2023). Similarly, disabled and neurodivergent SLT students continue to report discrimination in education and the workplace and this highlights the need to ensure that barriers to inclusion are removed (RCSLT, 2021c).

The profession requires a diverse workforce that reflects the communities that are served by it (RCSLT, 2022). It must therefore work to understand the current disparity of experience that students from all minoritised groups report as occurring on campus and placement (RCSLT, 2023a). Intersectionality, and how this may play out in the lived experience of the students on placement and in supervision must be considered. West's (2021) concept of inclusive leadership may provide the profession with key principles that enable an inclusive approach to supervision:

- Be self-aware and present in the moment, particularly in interactions with individuals that we perceive as 'other' or different from us.
- Consciously work harder to have regular contact and increase efforts to understand and empathise.
- First listen and then act upon what we learn, helping where we can.
- Consider reverse mentoring as an approach, to facilitate a mutual exchange whereby the student learns from your clinical experience and as an educator, you learn about the student's experience (West, 2021; Curtis et al., 2021).
- Where conflict occurs, defer judgement. Get curious, explore all perspectives to gain a shared perspective and understanding.
- Build trust by being consistent in your actions. Ask yourself are you consistently authentic, honest, open, appreciative, and compassionate?

Is sufficient value given to supervision?

- Regular supervision is recommended within the practice-based learning guidance (RCSLT, 2021b). When possible be clear from the start of placement what 'regular' supervision will look like in your work context and protect time.

- Assess and clarify the student's understanding of what supervision entails and manage expectations.
- Outline when supervision will take place throughout the placement. Even, if the day varies each week, or needs to be changed, having a plan will help the student to see that there are specific touch points where they can speak with their supervisor and discuss progress. This also gives the student opportunities to prepare for supervision.
- Where more than one practice educator is supporting students on the same placement, it may be beneficial for one practice educator to take responsibility for providing weekly professional supervision.
- Some trusts now have AHP placement leads who offer supervision or interprofessional supervision (where other student health professionals access group supervision). Find out whether this offer is available within your trust or your organisation. Ensure the student knows how to opt into this opportunity.

The student is doing well, is supervision necessary?

All students must have the opportunity to receive supervision (RCSLT, 2021b). Supervision will hopefully support students irrespective of their stage of professional development. Without regular supervision there is also a danger that educators can assume that students have capabilities that they have not yet developed. Bias can influence your decision making. You may find that you are working with a student who is excelling in their practice. Nevertheless, observing the student perspective, supervision remains an important learning tool. Everyone requires validation, opportunities to reflect on and extend their practice and for achievements to be celebrated. Again, supervision ensures this type of acknowledgement is an integral element of lifelong learning.

Perhaps, during supervision you discover that students are working exceptionally long days or evenings in order sustain the level of achievement that you are observing. Without exploring this working pattern, the students could be at risk of 'burn out'. Healthy work-life balance is essential for placement and beyond. Whilst being a lecturer I have worked with several students who have risked their mental health, sacrificing well-being in pursuit of perfection. Through supervision students can be supported to seek excellence positively and safely.

Concluding thoughts

This chapter discusses the role of supervision in SLT practice education. Points raised reflect my experience of supervision on placement, as a student, a practice educator and university lecturer. This chapter places supervision as central to student development, highlights the responsibilities of practice educators, as well as exploring how practice educators can best support SLT students and themselves whilst engaging in practice education. The student-educator relationship is a dynamic relationship that is nurtured in both the clinical context and under the influence of wider social, economic and political factors. Excellent supervision can be seen as an investigation into the student-educator relationship and insights shared in this chapter are offered to support practice educators with this exploration.

When working with students it is essential that we firstly remember our own position; the challenges and the privileges that inform who we are in all aspects of our practice, including practice education. We should not assume we know the background or current experiences that influence a student's ability to apply their knowledge and skill, or what might prevent engagement in any form of supervision. We must seek to understand, facilitate, teach and not judge. Assessment is a necessary part of education, a summary of an end point. Learning, with the support of great teachers is the journey. As a profession we must agree and give clarity to students about what to expect from supervision, giving clear demarcation between managerial and professional supervision.

References

Brown, B. (2018) *Daring to Lead*. London: Random House Penguin.

Baxter, S. (2004) Fit for Practice: New models for clinical placements, in Brumfitt, S. (2004) *Innovations in Professional Education For Speech and Language Therapy*. London: Whurr Publishers Ltd.

Clarke, A. Kessie, A. Ogunbanke, B. (2021) True to Ourselves. RCSLT Bulletin, January.

Curtis, S., Mozley, H., Langford, C., Hartland, J., Kelly, J. (2021) Challenging the deficit discourse in medical schools through reverse mentoring – Using discourse analysis to analysis to explore staff perceptions of underrepresented medical students. *BMJ Open,* 11: e054890. doi:10.1136/bmjopen-2021-054890

Dabiri, E. (2019) *Don't Touch My Hair*. London: Penguin Random House UK.

Geller, E. (2015) Using oneself as a vehicle for change in relational and reflective practice, in Fourie, R. J. (2015) *Therapeutic Processes for Communication Disorders: A Guide for Clinicians and Students*. Psychology Press.

Grant, A. (2023) Breaking free of stereotype threat with Claude Steele. Working Life with Adam Grant. Available at: https://podcasts.google.com/feed/aHR0cHM6Ly 9mZWVkcy5mZWVkYnVybmVyLmNvbS9Xb3JbGlmZVdpdGgBZGFtR3Jhbn Q/ episode/MTAwMDU5NjE3MDM2MA?ep=14 [Accessed 9 February 2023].

Gyimah, M., Azad, Z., Begum, S., Kapoor, A., Ville, L. Henderson, A., Dey, M. (2022) Broken Ladders: The myth of meritocracy for women of colour in the workplace. *The Fawcett Society & The Runnymede Trust*.

Harding, D. (2019) Practitioner Permeability and the resolution of practice uncertainties: A grounded theoretical perspective of supervision for Allied Health Professionals, s.l.: s.n.

HCPC (2022a) The benefits and outcomes of effective supervision. www.hcpc-uk.org/ standards/meeting-our-standards/supervision-leadership-and-culture/supervision/ the-benefits-and-outcomes-of-effective-supervision/ [Accessed 3 June 2022].

HCPC (2022b) Approaching supervision. www.hcpc-uk.co.uk/standards/meeting-our-standards/supervision-leadership-and-culture/supervision/approaching-supervision/ [Accessed 3 June 2022].

Kinouani, G. (2021) *Living While Black*. London: Penguin Random House UK.

Packer, M. (2023) Breakdown or breakthrough? in Malik, M. *A Vision from the Margin: Intersectional Insights on Navigating Diversity in Speech and Language Therapy*. Croydon: J & R Press Ltd.

RCSLT (2021a) Supervision Guidance. Available at: www.rcslt.org/members/deliv ering-quality-services/supervision/supervision-guidance/ [Accessed 18 September 2021].

RCSLT (2021b) Practice Based Learning Guidance: Main Guidance. Available at: www.rcslt.org/members/lifelong-learning/practice-based-learning/practice-based-learning-guidance/ [Accessed 11 December 2022].

RCSLT (2021c) Supporting Students with a Disability in the Workplace. Available at: www.rcslt.org/learning/diversity-inclusion-and-anti-racism/supporting-slts-with-disabilities-in-the-workplace/#section-1 [Accessed 11 December 2022].

RCSLT (2022) Strategic Vision 2022–2027. www.rcslt.org/news/the-rcslt-strategic-vision-2022-2027/ [Accessed 11 December 2022].

RCSLT (2023a) Analysing Diversity Equity and Inclusion in Speech and Language. www.rcslt.org/wp-content/uploads/2023/02/Anti-racism-survey-report-Feb-2023.pdf [Accessed 14 April 2023].

RCSLT (2023b) *Supervision Guidance*. Available at: www.rcslt.org/members/deliv ering-quality-services/supervision/supervision-guidance/#section-1 [Accessed 21 October 2023].

Snowdon, D., Sargeant, M., Williams, C., Maloney, S., Caspers K., Taylor, N. (2020) *Effective Clinical Supervision of Allied Health Professionals: A Mixed Methods Study*. BMC Health Services Research. https://doi.org/10.1186/s12913-019-4873-8

Steele, C. (1997) A Threat in the Air: How Stereotypes Shape Intellectual Identity and performance. *American Psychologist*, 52(6): 613–629.

Stokes, J. (2015) Supervision in speech and language therapy: Learning from other professions, in Stokes, J. and McCormick (eds) *Speech and Language Therapy: Challenging Received Wisdom*. Croydon: J & R Press

Spencer, M. and Healey, J. (2022) *Surviving Placement in Health and Social Care: A Student Handbook*, 2nd edn. London: Open University Press.

Tucker, K. (2023) An Exploration of Early-Stage Professional Identity Development: The Being and Becoming of First-Year Speech and Language Therapy Students. Available at: https://figshare.cardiffmet.ac.uk/articles/thesis/An_exploration_of_early-stage_professional_identity_development_The_being_and_becoming_of_first-year_speech_and_language_therapy_students/22665715/1 [Accessed 09 December 2023].

West, M. (2021) *Compassionate Leadership: Sustaining Wisdom, Humanity and Presence in Health and Social Care*. UK: The Swirling Leaf Press.

4

Insights into Supervision in SLT
Exploring the Experiences of Ethnic Minority Clinicians and Reflections on Continued Practice

Ilyeh Nahdi and Sahar Nashir

We write this chapter as women of ethnic minority backgrounds and explore racial topics as the prominent feature of our experiences. We are both speech and language therapists. Sahar has experience in the United Kingdom (UK) National Health Service (NHS) specialising in paediatric acquired brain injury. Ilyeh has worked with children with complex physical, learning and mental health needs in a secondary special school and the community. We are also experienced in delivering bespoke anti-racism training to fellow clinicians, educators and student speech and language therapists.

We cover themes that cross the intersectionalities of protected characteristic groups and the marginalised. However, the lack of discourse on the wellbeing of clinicians from ethnic minorities and the potential of supervision in this regard will be forefront. We draw upon discussions and data collated through the online platform *SLTea Time,* (2020a, 2020b, 2021a, 2021b) which seeks to prioritise topics of race within the speech and language therapy (SLT) narrative.

We met in 2020, alongside other passionate and active speech and language therapists from ethnic minority backgrounds to form *SLTea Time.* It was here that discussions on race, disparities and inequalities within our profession were showcased through social media platforms, tools which had proven highly useful in amplifying topics of importance during the height of the Black Lives Matter movement. *SLTea Time* grew and changed, becoming a space of support for ethnic minority speech and language therapists and students. The direction changed from emotionally motivated criticism

DOI: 10.4324/9781003301141-4

against the system to strategic actions for instigating change, mirroring the Black Lives Matter movement itself. Through this platform we were able to engage with anti-racism work, develop training courses and create a space for speech and language therapists from ethnic minority backgrounds to be part of the discourse.

Supervision occurs throughout SLT training and practice. In recent times, we suggest it has become imperative to oversee and nurture the supervision space with both a political and social lens. It has never been more crucial to address racial trauma and increase such dialogue within the SLT profession. Recent events, societal realities and the resurgence of political movements such as Black Lives Matter, have slowly moved team, service and organisational dialogues towards anti-racist practice. This includes greater inclusivity, representation and finding ways to reduce health inequality. Across SLT the pace of change in policy and practice differs greatly. While some people from ethnic minority groups have improving experiences, barriers to accessing supervision remain. Here we share some insights and possibilities for further progress.

When effective (Rothwell, Kehoe & Farook, 2021), supervision offers a space for reflecting on the uncertainties that arise in everyday practice. With this thinking, it is no longer imagined as an uninvolved space with the sole purpose of clinical problem solving, but as an active, holistic environment for effective development and the support of practitioners' mental health and wellbeing. Harding (2019) describes practitioners who have the skills necessary to utilise the space in this way as 'permeable'. They are self-aware, aware of and for others, awareness sharing, feedback-seeking, open to alternatives, critically attuned and ultimately willing to change. For example, if self-aware, one can recognise one's own uncertainties and perhaps reflect within supervision to assess gaps in knowledge for development. We welcome this as a direct framework to addressing areas such as clinician bias within SLT.

The Royal College of Speech and Language Therapists, (RCSLT, 2017) describes supervision as managerial supervision or professional supervision and differentiates both from professional support. Our main focus here is professional supervision. This form of supervision is highlighted as a way of discussing clinical and non-clinical professional issues in non-judgemental environments and is often provided by another speech and language therapist without line-management responsibility (RCSLT, 2017). The Health and Care Professions Council (HCPC) outline supervision as a requirement for professionals who are regulated by the body, including speech and language therapists. More recently, HCPC guidelines (2022) were revised to involve more focus on clinicians' awareness of the impact of culture, equality and diversity on practice, and to place importance on practice being inclusive for service users. As we discuss supervision and race within SLT in this chapter we draw on the impacts of missing knowledge, dialogue and research. Additionally, we suggest continued actions that may benefit the experience of supervision for ethnic minority speech and language therapists.

Speech and language therapy: the UK context

With a steady emergence and focus on diversity and inclusion, it is essential that supervision reflects cultural teaching, acknowledges bias and provides a space for honest conversation between individuals who are open to receiving feedback and learning about others. Cultural responsiveness must be integrated to allow others to learn from and relate to people of their own culture and of other cultures. Practitioners' experiences as both supervisors and supervisees begin in training and experiences within educational settings/university which can influence confidence and competence in delivering and receiving inclusive supervision. Cultural responsiveness must begin in those early experiences.

RCSLT 2019–2020 figures on ethnic diversity (RCSLT, 2019) showed that 75% of the total population of speech and language therapists identified as white, with 9% being unaccounted for, 3% identified as Black, 9% Asian, 3% identified as mixed and 1% 'other'. Drawing on Harding (2019), if supervision is imagined as permeable practitioners sharing alternative experiences and resolutions, there must also be awareness of how this can be achieved when one or more of these practitioners are from ethnic minority backgrounds. Different and shared perspectives, lived experiences and cultural contexts play a significant role in how situations are approached and resolved and cannot be dismissed when attempting to create a secure space for personal and professional development.

The potential of supervision for ethnic minorities

The first priority for a health system should be fostering an inclusive and supportive environment that facilitates personal and professional growth. Clinicians from diverse backgrounds provide valuable insight and creativity stemming from unique perspectives and experiences. Given that ethnic minority individuals may encounter specific challenges, wider experiences or cultural barriers in their practice, a culturally responsive supervisory relationship can enable them to discuss these issues openly and safely. This, in turn, promotes the development of culturally competent care, which is vital in addressing health disparities and improving patient outcomes across diverse populations.

Supervisors can provide guidance and constructive feedback to help professionals refine their skills, gain confidence, and better understand the intricacies of their profession. Encouraging opportunities for supervision with experienced practitioners from minority backgrounds who may have faced similar challenges, can empower ethnic minority professionals to navigate their careers more effectively. Furthermore, this mentorship can play a crucial role in fostering a sense of belonging and resilience, helping these professionals feel valued and supported within the workplace. Equally, we suggest that supervision with, for and from ethnic minority perspectives can contribute to a more inclusive and diverse healthcare environment. By actively supporting and nurturing the development of professionals from various backgrounds, healthcare organisations can work towards greater representation within their workforce. This increased diversity not only helps to break down barriers and challenge biases, but also brings a wider range of perspectives and experiences to the table. Ultimately, this results in improved decision-making, better communication, and a more comprehensive understanding of the needs of diverse patient populations.

Barriers to supervision for clinicians from ethnic minority backgrounds

Barriers and facilitators of supervision are recognised (Rothwell, Kehoe & Farook, 2021; Kilminster & Jolly, 2000; Snowdon et al., 2020) but there is limited discussion of racial or cultural barriers which we now explore with reference to our and others' experiences.

Racial trauma

Experiences of racism, discrimination and microaggressions, both in and out of the workplace, take a toll on an individual's physical and mental health (Spanierman, Clark & Kim, 2021). Additionally, the experience many ethnic minority families go through in the process of migration from war-torn countries to the West, weighs heavily on their community's collective wellbeing and perception of self. Oppressive conditions, objectification by the system and lack of equal access to services for black and ethnic minority communities psychologically damages those who experience it, resulting in racial trauma. In *SLTea Time* (2021a) we explored this topic in depth. We discussed the ongoing effects of racism, racial bias and exposure to racist abuse directly or indirectly and the impact of media characterisations that diminish a person's sense of worth.

This topic warrants a publication of its own. It is relevant in this chapter because racial trauma can present similarly to Post-Traumatic Stress Disorder (Butts, 2002). Many health professionals are navigating such complex emotions and anxieties daily. This is an important consideration if supervisors are to create a safe space and trusting relationship for effective supervision (Rothwell, Kehoe & Farook 2021). This is made difficult by the way the impact of racial trauma manifests itself. Internalised devaluation, distorted sense of self and 'psychological homelessness' (Negy et al., 2014) resulting in a distorted sense of home and belonging, in turn make it difficult to feel truly safe anywhere and hesitant to trust those assigned to protect.

The student experience

SLTea Time data indicated that 65% *of* 75 speech and language therapists and students had sadly experienced microaggressions. Racial microaggressions are defined as commonplace verbal or behavioural indignities, whether intentional or unintentional, which communicate hostile, derogatory, or negative racial insults (Sue, 2010). In a discussion between practising speech and language therapists, SLT students, and a PhD researcher investigating hate crime and microaggressions experienced by international students in the UK, *SLTea Time* (2020b) explored the meaning of microaggressions, identifying them and responding to these within the workplace/university, particularly as ethnic minority group members navigating the healthcare space. *SLTea Time* also spoke to guests who felt more confident and able to raise awareness of such issues. This has informed our ideas about how collaboration can enable story-sharing and hopefully increase the sharing of concerns during supervision. Supervisors may have a significant and key role here in supporting clinicians in replicating this environment as well as finding which methods work for their supervisee in sharing information and communicating issues and difficulties faced. There may also be scope here for group and peer supervision opportunities, where conversations are widened.

Through *SLTea Time* we heard of negative experiences of discrimination in places of work, universities, healthcare settings, community settings and hospitals. Some experienced directly from peers, colleagues, service users and some from strangers or less familiar people. Many students explained feelings of long-term anxiety, low confidence and reports of lower self-esteem which discouraged them from speaking up, seeking support and raising incidents to higher management and/or university tutors. These experiences mirrored newly qualified therapist experiences in many ways; with similarities in the ways in which microaggressions and racial abuse left long-lasting impacts on physical and emotional health. For some, the experiences were overshadowed by the demands of training and practising as a clinician. Other students shared that they decided to leave the profession, sought routes into more inclusive professions or away from healthcare where they felt better represented and could share their experiences free from fear of potential discipline.

Sadly, many students reported they had experienced incidents with trusted educators and practice mentors and supervisors; to which no further action was taken. Reflecting on this, we suggest these experiences raise an additional issue of how the relationship within supervision is pivotal in creating and nurturing conversations that address discrimination, racial abuse and the impacts on our professional and personal lives. Additionally, we wonder how equipped practice educators and supervisors are to support this category of uncertainty. There is a role for both supervisor and supervisee here in shared empathy of experience. *SLTea Time* (2020b) also addressed the cathartic experience of sharing and feeling protected, as if it was not 'just in our heads' or not something we had misread or misunderstood. Instead, we acknowledge that the more inclusive supervisors and educators we had met and learned from provided us with reassurance and recognised negative experiences and emotions. We have found Ibrahim's Anti-Racist Model (Ibrahim, 2020), explains this well. This framework, created at the height of the Black Lives Matter movement, describes 'Fear', 'Growth' and 'Learning' zones, alongside statements indicative of each zone. These include avoiding hard questions in the Fear Zone, being vulnerable about own biases and knowledge gaps in the Learning Zone and in the Growth Zone, sitting

Table 4.1 Indicative statements in relation to zones of becoming anti-racist

Becoming anti-racist		
Fear zone	Learning zone	Growth zone
• I deny Racism is a problem. • I avoid hard questions. • I strive to be comfortable. • I talk to others who look & think like me.	• I recognise racism is a present & current problem. • I seek out questions that make me uncomfortable. • I understand my own privilege in ignoring Racism. • I educate myself about race & structural Racism. • I am vulnerable about my own biases & knowledge gaps. • I listen to others who think & look differently than me.	• I identify how I may unknowingly benefit from Racism. • I promote & advocate for policies & leaders that are Anti-Racist • I sit with my discomfort. • I speak out when I see Racism in action. • I educate my peers how Racism harms our profession. • I don't let mistakes deter me from being better. • I yield positions of power to those otherwise marginalised. • I surround myself with others who think & look differently than me.

Ibrahim (2020)

in discomfort and listening without becoming defensive. These statements, summarised in Table 4.1, allow clinicians and individuals to focus on self-development in each area.

In SLT there may be additional barriers in supervision spaces. For example, as a relatively smaller profession with even smaller specialisms there can be overlap between management and professional or clinical supervision and variation in supervision training experiences. We encourage teams to broaden experiences of supervisor training and development to allow more focus on models such as Ibrahim's (2020). With reference to permeability (Harding, 2019), supervisor training should encourage self-reflection and discussion around positionality and for supervisors to be alert to their own influences, position and assumptions, and the potential for these to differ from the supervisees'. Having resources, such as regular use of theoretical frameworks and profession-wide discussions may enable supervisors to seek feedback from their supervisees.

The supervisor and the supervisee

Snowdon et al. (2020) suggest that supervisor skills and attributes facilitate constructive supervisory relationships. In our experience, the skills and attributes required by either party in the supervision process when one or both are from ethnic minority backgrounds are not always so easily defined or recognised.

Within working relationships between supervisee and supervisor, there are visible signs of power imbalance. Power for the supervisor due to their title or seniority as examples. The supervisor holds many different responsibilities beyond clinical practice. This could include performance rating, promotion, recognition, praise or critical evaluation of work and development. We suggest that differences in power should be acknowledged, reviewed and discussed openly.

Rothwell, Kehoe & Farook (2021) identify 'successful' supervisors as empathetic, respectful and genuine, combined with tolerance, self-knowledge and clinical expertise. Supervisees may naturally recognise their responsibilities within the context of their own role. They may also feel pressured to say or do things to fulfil their duties or imitate skills learned from their mentor or supervisor. In our experience there can be occasions where the opposite occurs and things may be left undetailed. As Sweeney and Creaner (2014) report, the overall quality of the supervisory relationship is a significant element in nondisclosure. Difference and power within supervision is inevitable. Therefore, the way in which characteristics and lived experiences are shared to create a mutual understanding is vital.

We argue that the impacts of cultural norms, roles and rules might dictate our supervision experiences. For example, many cultural norms have deeper entrenched rules for respecting authority, use of language in the workplace or educational settings and expectations of supervision/practice. Fong (1994) describes the importance of establishing a base of trust and empathy by clearly outlining expectations of supervision and an open discussion about similarities and differences from a very early stage. There is a real importance for self-reflective skills and at a fundamental level for openness, respect and honesty. Boundaries should be kept and held, with confidentiality and integrity at the core. When thinking about service users and clinical cases, there is an opportunity to strive to utilise supervision as a space to challenge practice, with honest feedback and to draw on shared experiences.

Our experiences and those of our podcast guests and followers indicate barriers in establishing a safe space for supervisee and/or supervisor, such as allocated time (or lack thereof), lack of clinical or cultural knowledge or negative prior supervision experiences. For many, early negative placement and/or university experiences may contribute to feeling unsafe, unheard and at higher risk for discipline. Schen & Greenlee (2018) explain the ethno-cultural differences between supervisor and supervisee can create feelings of insecurity which may lead to extra attentiveness to professional standards, guidelines and over-criticising work. Allyship is relevant here and should not be underestimated in supervisory relationships. Arguably being able to also advocate for each other's needs creates stronger and healthier supervision experiences; ones in which both parties involved can share personal experiences, and clinical cases with a more positive framework of how culture, race, ethnicity, age and language are therapeutic strengths. We advocate for the importance of allyship, particularly as through *SLTea Time*, we have observed the impact of wider groups of individuals supporting our work.

Supervision within the political system

We both argue that the impact of systemic policies directly relating to therapists from ethnic minorities must be considered. We reflect on the UK Consider Prevent Programme (GOV UK, 2011), a counter-radicalisation and counter-terrorism strategy in which it is the duty of healthcare workers to report individuals they suspect are susceptible to radicalisation based on elusive 'pre-criminal' risk factors. Muslims of Middle Eastern or Asian descent are by far the largest representation reported to Prevent, which ties to decades of mainstream media representation of Muslims as the archetype candidates as terrorists. The racialisation of 'threat to national security' in public consciousness gives prejudice institutional legitimacy (Younis & Jadhav, 2020). For Muslims, undertaking the Prevent training necessary to work as a healthcare practitioner can be traumatising and isolating, prompting constant feelings of guilt, shame, monitoring and the necessity to prove oneself as the deviation from the 'norm'.

We see this as relevant in supervision, as a supervisee may bring these emotions to supervision as a direct result of the system that is offering it. Whilst the intention to create a safe and protected supervision environment is commendable this is impossible without an understanding of the context and circumstances the supervisee is entering the space from. The supervisee's uncertainties may arise from experiences that the supervisor cannot even contemplate without prior thought, discussion and education. Without these, supervision transforms instead to a tick box exercise in which shallow concerns, most likely clinical, are explored and resolved, as necessary for organisational development. The supervisee will leave the space, perhaps slightly more clinically proficient, whilst continuing to navigate their profession with distrust, fear and uncertainty.

Possible foundations for safe supervision

Next, we draw on some of our own experiences and reflections to provide possibilities for more inclusive supervision.

Promoting self-reflection

Critical reflection is a core part of speech and language therapists' development. Ilyeh reflects on her early experiences in delivering 'reflective practice' training for teachers and assistants:

I was sometimes surprised that colleagues seemed less familiar with this concept. However, the same colleagues responded positively to the idea of critical reflection when introduced to it and I observed that although it was sometimes a struggle, it supported them to move from subjective to more objective problem solving and fostered a willingness to change personally and professionally. Reflecting further on those experiences, something else occurs to me. My exposure to critical reflection in my professional training is part of the story but there is an added dimension which I suggest arises from my experiences as a person from a minority group. Where others might struggle to grasp the concept of a reflective process and repeatedly bring subjective experiences to the table that require a high level of support to remove themselves from, I found myself comfortable with dissociation as someone who has had to repeatedly do so within my career in order to fit into the 'typical' projection of what a therapist should be.

Self-reflection and self-awareness did not seem to be something that colleagues were utilising readily. In contrast, marginalisation results in unavoidable confrontation of one's 'self'. Being different to the 'norm' prompts tendencies towards constant reflection and self-awareness. Society reminds us of it every day. There is a system and health professional archetype that we, the marginalised, do not fit in by default and therefore we must reflect on how to mould into this acceptable version of ourselves that can function in Western healthcare systems. Alongside feeling the impact of social injustice first hand, we are driven to pursue social change. As a result of these critical reflection skills, we are constantly imagining and reimagining a healthcare system that is relevant to our communities and welcomes us to the workforce as equals. An unacknowledged self-awareness gap can often exist between an ethnic minority supervisee and a supervisor in the dominant SLT demographic, and vice versa. Closing this gap through the development of self-reflection skills and bias-awareness training is vital in ensuring that both members of the supervision experience are entering the space on an equitable foundation.

Training (a focus on self-reflection and positionality)

Ensuring that colleagues are appropriately equipped with the tools to access and create supervision spaces must be at the forefront of our priorities as healthcare professionals. This is particularly true when colleagues are from diverse ethnic backgrounds. This has been a focus of our work, using *SLTea Time* to form connections with NHS organisations and universities for the purpose of delivering such training. With frameworks, such as the Social GGRRAAACCEEESSS Model (Burnham,1992, 2013; Roper-Hall, 1998) in Figure 4.1, we have developed training that invites speech and language therapists to reflect on their positionality within their social and professional contexts. Once identification has been made, they are invited to reflect on which intersections hold power. Such a training may seem obvious yet unless explicitly given time, this level of thinking and application to one's career is not often made. Feedback received from these training sessions is overwhelmingly positive (SLTea Time, 2021a), particularly with student speech and language therapists who perhaps feel more confident in making changes to their practice before the creation of longer-term clinical habits and considerations of self-reflection, bias and clinical decision making.

Social GRACES

Power Relations in Society
Values held by people in relation to social difference
Potential to devalue according to difference

- Gender
- Geography
- Race
- Religion
- Age
- Accent
- Appearance
- Physical
- Intellectual
- Social
- Abilities
- Affiliation
- Emotional

- Spirituality
- Sexuality
  - Sexual Orientation
  - Sexual Expression
- Size
- Ethnicity
- Colour
- Class
- Culture

Mnemonic Acronym to prompt therapeutic focus on the influence of social difference

© Alison Roper-Hall

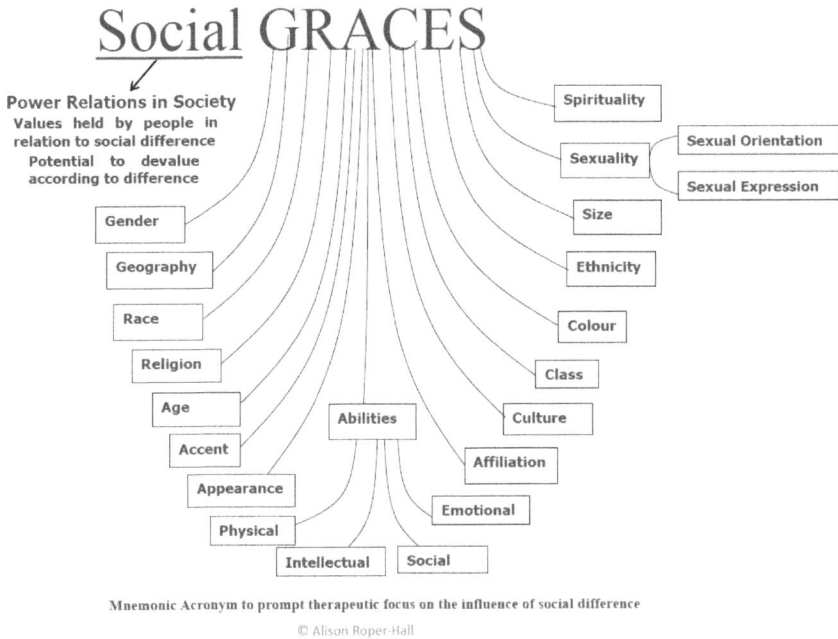

Figure 4.1 The Social GGRRAAAACCEEESSS Model with permission of Alison Roper-Hall

(Burnham, 1992, 2013; Roper-Hall, 1998)

Drawing on a solution-focused approach

Sahar draws on her practice experiences of solution-focused approaches in which the supervisee and the client are key partners in the process of change and identifying what is working well (Dewane, 2015, Walsh, 2013). She reflects on work with service users in which feedback, areas of development and reflections on practice were shared at points of discharge from SLT. Sahar suggests that with a solution-focused approach and consistent co-production, many aspects of culturally sensitive and inclusive practice can be woven into SLT and supervision. This type of supervision focuses on the future, repetition of positive progress and what works, with the key focus being on *solution* rather than examining issues or problems. This may provide space for authentic conversations around wider considerations, such as a client's religion, ethnicity, race, culture and their language or communication goals as well as ways practitioners can learn more about differences within the populations they serve. Solution-focused approaches in supervision can allow identification of what is working well for us as practitioners and for our service users, encouraging open conversations about strengths and skills. For example, 'what are some of the best things about being in your shoes and how can you use this in practice?'. It highlights successes, uses scaling but also uses silence to support the generation of ideas and deeper reflective thought. Being solution-focused may be one of the easiest approaches which could use more widely to benefit professional and personal development and the work delivered in diverse communities.

Psychological safety

Supervision spaces must create a safe environment for open and honest disclosure of feelings, emotions and reflections on client work (Pelling, Barletta & Armstrong, 2009). We, therefore, suggest that psychological safety must be a more explicit priority in the workplace and supervision context. It could be viewed as a sense of humility. Clinician humility has been described in medical care as positively predicting patient satisfaction, trust and therapy outcomes (Huynh & Dicke-Bohmann, 2020). Cultural humility when practised regularly within supervision spaces may also be key to establishing positive experiences and having a "growth and learning" mindset. Akin to the concept of life-long cultural competency learning, this is being on a journey rather than a 'tick-box compliance' activity.

Being more open-minded and compassionate includes celebrating others for challenging the 'status quo' and using critical frameworks that examine race, culture, linguistic difference and SLT practice. It may mean encouraging learning from trial and error in non-judgemental ways and exploring how team members communicate concerns about processes that are not working. This could lead clinicians to feel more adaptable and confident when thinking of change. This safety can enable team inclusion and team diversity, whilst encouraging and celebrating the many benefits that may arise from experiences, knowledge and backgrounds that would not be possible if our peers and service users are unable to share and listen intentionally to each other. We must acknowledge the experiences of others where they have felt unsafe such as repeated experiences of trauma, racial abuse, microaggressions, discrimination and how the supervisory space could exacerbate such issues.

In healthcare, additional inclusive spaces enable 'speaking up', for example, the NHS Freedom to Speak Up Programme (NHS, 2023) established following the Francis Report (Francis, 2015). Arguably, it is increasingly possible for supervisors to access support and guidance from such programmes and from equality and diversity leads, in organisational where these are established.

Concluding thoughts

We conclude this chapter with strong reference to the missing gaps in training, research and knowledge in the conversations around race and supervision. We envision this as a starting point for continued progress. We acknowledge the influence of training within SLT practice and the impact of utilising more inclusive frameworks and approaches to enable the roles of both supervisor and supervisee, when either one or both come from ethnic minority backgrounds. We reflect on experiences of delivering training to NHS trusts, peers and universities. There has been much positive change when focussing on reflection, positionality and introspection as the foundation of effective supervision. There is a need for examination of supervision for ethnic minority practitioners on a deeper level and training for colleagues in the current workforce, which we acknowledge requires additional research and policy change.

SLTea Time has enabled many discussions, initiatives and processes, which we feel is a positive step for continued development and change, from students to clinicians and those in academia. We argue these discussions can be replicated in supervision with the appropriate resources for emotional support, particularly for students and clinicians who may have experienced racism and discrimination. Systemic approaches can support us in asking peers the right questions and developing introspective skills within clinical practice and supervision. There is something to add here about the power of platforms like *SLTea Time* as spaces for honest and open discussion and also as catalysts for change and action. This is not a task for those of ethnic minority background alone, but a collective shift in the attitudes and discourse of the profession as a whole. Each and every clinician has responsibility in ensuring they are fully equipped in delivering and receiving safe supervision as part of their practice.

The idea of permeability in supervision is vital in the discourse of the wellbeing of ethnic minority speech and language therapists and students. This involves cultivating an openness to learning, self-reflection, and a willingness to adapt to new ideas and experiences. This process requires us to be receptive to feedback, actively listen to the perspectives of others, and embrace diverse viewpoints. At the time of writing this chapter, the Council of Deans of Health (2023) published 'Anti-racism in AHP Education: Building an Inclusive Environment'. We echo its recommendations, particularly for facilitation of safe spaces, for both students and speech and language therapists in practice and supervision. As described, this involves incorporating critical reflection by both supervisor and supervisee, to allow growth and development. It requires honest conversation as well as effective and appropriate materials and resources.

By acknowledging existing biases and continually examining assumptions, the flexibility needed to grow as professionals is possible. This growth, in turn, facilitates more effective, empathetic, and culturally sensitive care, ultimately enhancing the overall quality of practice and population well-being. We argue that everyone has a role in challenging racism, rethinking frameworks, and continuing to ensure supervision in SLT evolves accordingly. We warmly invite others within the profession and beyond to continue this discussion, contribute to research and make prioritised efforts for the development of clinical practice.

References

Burnham, J. (1992). Approach, Method, Technique: Making Distinctions and Creating Connections. *Human Systems: The Journal of Systemic Consultation and Management,* 3(1), 3–26.

Burnham, J. (2013). Developments in Social GGRRAAACCEEESSS: Visible-invisible, Voiced-unvoiced. In I. Krause (ed.), *Cultural Reflexivity.* London: Karnac

Butts, H. F. (2002). The black mask of humanity: racial/ethnic discrimination and post-traumatic stress disorder. *Journal of American Academic Psychiatry Law,* 30(3), 336–339.

Council of Deans of Health. (2023). Report: Anti Racism in AHP Education: Building an Inclusive Environment. Retrieved from: www.councilofdeans.org.uk/2023/04/council-of-deans-of-health-release-new-report-anti-racism-in-ahp-education-building-an-inclusive-environment/

Dewane, C. J. (2015). Solution-Focused Supervision: A Go-to Approach. *Social Work Today,* 15, 24–25.

Fong, M. L. (1994). Multicultural Issues in Supervision. *ERIC Digest,* 4, 1–3.

Francis, R. (2015) Freedom to Speak Up: An Independent Review into Creating an Open and Honest Reporting Culture in the NHS. Available online at: http://freedom

tospeakup.org.uk/wp-content/uploads/2014/07/F2SU_web.pdf [Last accessed 08.02.24]/

GOV UK (2011) Prevent Strategy. Available online at: https://www.gov.uk/govern ment/publications/prevent-strategy-2011 [Last accessed: 08.02.24].

Harding, D. (2019). *Practitioner Permeability and the Resolution of Practice Uncertainties: Grounded Theoretical Perspective of Supervision for Allied Health Professionals.* (As part of PhD thesis), St George's, University of London. Available online at: https://eprints.kingston.ac.uk/id/eprint/43854/6/Harding-D-43854.pdf Last accessed: 08.02.24

Health and Care Professions Council (HCPC), 2022. Equality, diversity and inclusion. Available online at: www.hcpc-uk.org/standards/standards-of-proficiency/reviewing-the-standards-of-proficiency/equality-diversity-and-inclusion/

Huynh, H. P., and Dicke-Bohmann, A. (2020). Humble Doctors, Healthy Patients? Exploring the Relationships between Clinical Humility and Patient Satisfaction, Trust and Health Status. *Patient Educ Couns*, 103(1), 173–179.

Ibrahim, A. M. (2020). Becoming Anti-Racist: A Framework. Model downloaded from: www.surgeryredesign.com/current

Kilminster, S. M., and Jolly, B. C. (2000). Effective Supervision in Clinical Practice Settings: A Literature Review. *Med Educ*, 34, 827–840. doi:10.1046/j.1365-2923.2000.00758.xpmid

Negy, C., Reig-Ferrer, A., Gaborit, M., and Ferguson, C. J. (2014). Psychological Homelessness and Enculturative Stress among US-Deported Salvadorans: A Preliminary Study with a Novel Approach. *J Immigrant Minority Health*, 16, 1278–1283: https://doi.org/10.1007/s10903-014-0006-y

NHS (2023) Freedom to Speak Up. Available online at: www.england.nhs.uk/ourwork/freedom-to-speak-up/ [Last accessed: 08.02.24].

Pelling, N., Barletta, J., and Armstrong, P. (2009). *The Practice of Clinical Supervision.* Australia: Bowen Hills.

Roper-Hall, A. (1998). Working Systemically with Older People and their Families who Have 'Come to Grief'. In P. Sutcliffe, G. Tufnell and U. Cornish (eds), *Working with the Dying and Bereaved: Systemic Approaches to Therapeutic Work.* London: Macmillan.

Rothwell, C., Kehoe, A., and Farook, S.F. (2021). Enablers and Barriers to Effective Clinical Supervision in the Workplace: A Rapid Evidence Review. *BMJ Open Journal*, 11, e052929. doi:10.1136/bmjopen-2021-052929

Royal College of Speech and Language Therapists, RCSLT. (2017). Supervision for Speech and Language Therapists. Retrieved from: www.rcslt.org/wp-content/uploads/media/docs/delivering-quality-services/supervision-summary-for-speech-and-language-therapists.pdf

Royal College of Speech and Language Therapists, RCSLT. (2019). Diversity and ethnicity figures in the United Kingdom. Retrieved from: www.rcslt.org/members/speech-and-language-therapy/careers-promotion-and-diversity/careers-fast-facts/#section-4

Schen, C. R., and Greenlee, A. (2018). Race in Supervision: Let's Talk About It. *Psychodynamic Psychiatry*, 46(1), 1–21.

SLTea Time (July 2020a) 'University and Student Experience'. Podcast available online at: EP 1.3 | University and Student Experience | SLTea Time [Last Accessed 28.12.23].

SLTea Time (Nov 2020b) 'Microaggressions'. Podcast available online at: EP 2.4 | Microaggressions | SLTea Time [Last Accessed 28.12.23].

SLTea Time (Feb 2021a) 'Trauma'. Podcast available online at: EP 03.01 | Trauma | SLTea Time [Last Accessed 28.12.23].

SLTea Time (Aug 2021b) ' "Supervision". Podcast available online at: EP 3.2 | Supervision | SLTea Time [Last Accessed 28.12.23].

Snowdon, D. A., Sargent, M., Williams, C. M., Maloney, S., Caspers, K., and Taylor, N. F. (2020) Effective Clinical Supervision of Allied Health Professionals: A Mixed Methods Study. *BMC Health Serv Res*, 20, 1–11. doi:10.1186/s12913-019-4873-8

Spanierman, L. B., Clark, A. D., and Kim, Y. (2021). Reviewing Racial Microaggressions Research: Documenting Experiences, Harmful Sequelae and Resistance Strategies. *Sage Journals*, 16(5).

Sue, D. W. (2010). *Microaggressions in Everyday Life: Race, Gender and Sexual Orientation*. London: John Wiley & Sons.

Sweeney, J., and Creaner, M. (2014). What's Not Being Said? Recollections of Non-disclosure in Clinical Supervision while in Training. *British Journal of Guidance and Counselling*, 42(2), 211–224.

Walsh, J. (2013). *Theories For Direct Social Work Practice*. Belmont, CA: Thomson.

Younis, T., and Jadhav, S. (2020), Islamophobia in the National Health Service: An Ethnography of Institutional Racism in PREVENT's Counter-Radicalisation Policy. *Sociol Health Illn*, 42, 610–626. https://doi.org/10.1111/1467-9566.13047

5 Establishing Supervision Practices
One Manager's Journey

Dawn Leoni

Throughout my career, I have been inspired, encouraged, and motivated by the wisdom and support of my professional supervisors. When I reflect, I see the golden threads of supervision shining like a web, stretching me when I needed stretching; acting like a cradle to hold me when the going was tough, all the while keeping me safe and stable when the strong winds of the National Health Service (NHS) blew the web. Now in an NHS management role, I am committed to embedding a culture of robust supervision[1] within the department. My aspiration is for my colleagues to experience the wonders to be discovered though their own supervision practices. It is from this perspective that I write this chapter, for the consideration of other health care leaders.

Here I share an eight-year journey that our speech and language therapy (SLT) service has been on to embed robust professional supervision practices within a team of around 150 staff. I will reflect from a project management and change management perspective and aspire to motivate other organisations to strengthen their professional supervision practices, by benefitting from the learning within the chapter.

I will use Kotter's Eight stage process for leading change (Kotter, 1996, 2018) to retrospectively reflect (Figure 5.1). I should be clear at this point that at the commencement of the supervision project, the plan was not approached from this perspective, but reviewing the project using Kotter's constructs has provided valuable insight for leading future change.

DOI: 10.4324/9781003301141-5

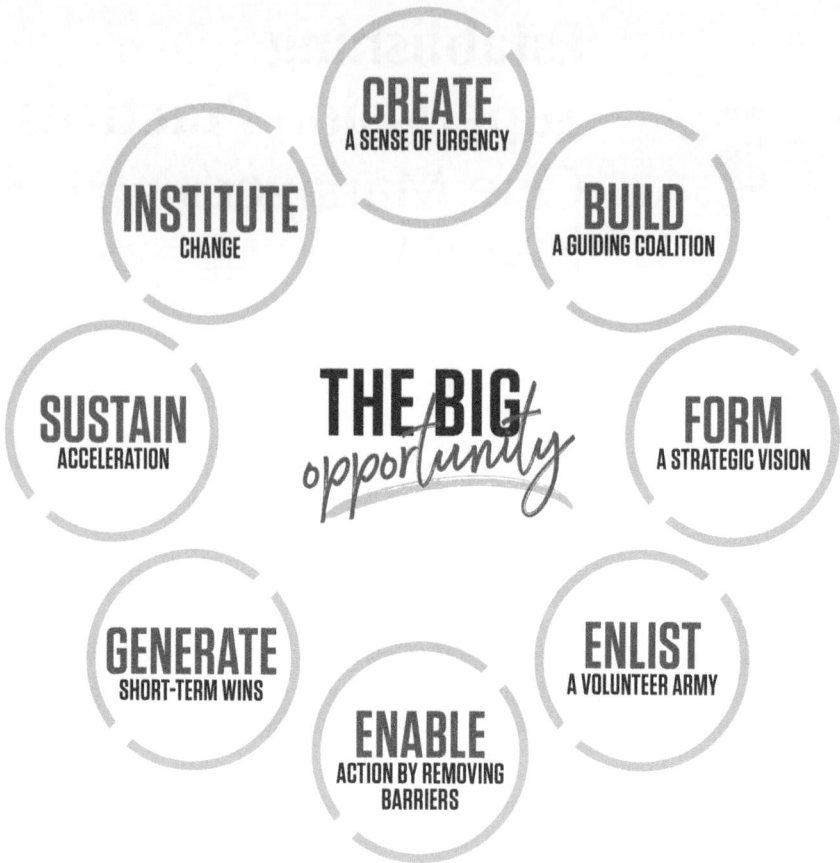

CREATE
A SENSE OF URGENCY

INSTITUTE
CHANGE

BUILD
A GUIDING COALITION

SUSTAIN
ACCELERATION

THE BIG
opportunity

FORM
A STRATEGIC VISION

GENERATE
SHORT-TERM WINS

ENABLE
ACTION BY REMOVING
BARRIERS

ENLIST
A VOLUNTEER ARMY

Figure 5.1

Background and context of the supervision project

When we started considering supervision practices in 2014, there were professional guidelines available (RCSLT, 2012; HCPC 2016; AWSLTMC, 2008) from which the department had created a local professional supervision protocol. These were outdated, and there were known variances in practice. The guidance provided clarity on the frequency, content, and documentation for supervision. However, the supervision provision lacked governance; for example, there was no method of monitoring participation in supervision, understanding the quality of the supervision provided, or ensuring the impact of the supervision on patient care or staff wellbeing within work. At this time, the guidance from the professional body lacked the detail that became available in later editions (RCSLT, 2017) and was therefore open to individual interpretation. There was evidence of inappropriate professional supervision practice within the teams, for example a specialist clinician accessing regular "professional supervision" to support her work with a person with aphasia from a non-registered clinical assistant who was herself untrained in supervision practices or stroke rehabilitation.

Kotter's Step 1: Creating a sense of urgency

Kotter outlines the need to create a sense of urgency, and on reflection for us, this took place by conducting a survey of supervision practices. The findings of this survey were stark. An extremely small number of clinicians were accessing supervision at all. There were different perceptions and views of what supervision was; some clinicians were supervisors to many people, and some were supervising no one. There were variances across staff grades, with more junior therapists, newly qualified therapists (UK NHS band 5) reporting greater access to supervision, but more specialist clinicians (UK NHS band 7 and above in the organisation) reporting lowest access due to struggles finding a supervisor within the same clinical specialism. There were variances linked to geographical locality and clinical specialism. However, unanimously, the clinicians who had participated in the survey placed a high value on supervision. This juxtaposition was puzzling: therapists valued professional supervision, and yet were not consistently accessing it. The reason for this was unclear - was it custom and practice, culture within teams, lack of understanding of the importance of supervision, lack of training for supervisors and supervisees, lack of time and conflicting demands on clinician's time?

In Kotter's terms, the findings from this survey provided sufficient evidence of the window of opportunity to act. Creating a sense of urgency is crucial to gaining cooperation to engage in change, and Kotter provides a well-recognised consideration of complacency in organisations as a barrier to successful change. The findings exposed the reality that beneath the professional guidance and local protocols, the reality of the supervision culture and practice was falling short of expectations. Sharing this data with senior managers, and staff, allowed us to have honest conversations and expose the need for action. The motivation for change was evident in the high value therapists assigned to professional supervision, and the momentum for change increased as supervision was discussed within teams.

Kotter's Step 2: Build a guiding coalition

This stage is described as the nerve centre of the change process (Kotter, 2018, p13). It describes the importance of selecting the right team to drive change. The team should represent various levels within the organisational structure, from diverse functions, and localities, and whose members demonstrate commitment to the change required.

Having recognised the requirement for change in supervision practices, approval was given by the senior leadership team to set up a supervision working group to lead a service improvement project. As I reflect on the team

Characteristic	Description	Our team
Position power	Ensure management representation within the team to ensure that progress cannot easily be blocked	One senior operational manager Two senior governance leads
Expertise	A range of points of view are represented to enable informed decision-making	Two adult SLTs Three paediatric SLTs Representation from each geographical locality
Credibility	Team to include members with good reputations who will be taken seriously by other employees	All group members were felt to have demonstrated credibility and leadership within their working environments
Leadership	Sufficient leaders within the team to drive change	

Figure 5.2 Kotter's key characteristics of a change team applied retrospectively to our project team

(Kotter 1996, p. 57)

we assembled to take forward the next phase of the project, I recognise some key concepts from Kotter's guidance about building a guiding coalition.

Kotter outlines the need for a coalition to have trust and to develop a common goal, which can be achieved by regular events, discussion, and shared activities. Our initial meetings involved sharing experiences, perceptions, and observations of professional supervision practices. It unfolded that there were a range of professional supervision models in use. Peer supervision and group supervision were cited, but with limited definition of what the groups involved or the learning outcomes were for participants.

We reviewed professional and regulatory guidelines, from the RCSLT, other allied health professional bodies, nursing and midwifery, organisational guidance, and our departmental protocols. We found a range of differences in the delivery of supervision including direct supervision models, peer support, management supervision and professional supervision. There was a lack of clarity on what training should be provided to enable a clinician to become a supervisor, how competency in supervision is demonstrated, measured, and maintained. Consideration needed to be made regarding frequency, documentation, selection of supervisor, allocation of supervisees and how line management could have oversight of the supervision arrangement. We were keen to have consistency of approach if a supervisory relationship broke down, was not considered supportive, or if professional practice safety issues had been raised.

A common theme that emerged was the abstract concept of motivation (and conversely, complacency) within the staff group to participate in supervision. How could we motivate and inspire our teams to invest and participate in supervision as well as ensure that the systems and processes were put in place to support robust supervision practices? How could we ensure that registered professionals could meet the standards outlined by the regulatory and professional bodies? This review took place in 2015, at a time when professional bodies were in the process of developing revised guidance, and as such, it is possible that our organisational practices were mirrored in other SLT services.

Kotter's Step 3: Form a strategic vision and initiatives

Vision, according to Kotter, is essential in creating a picture of the future. Providing vision and direction with a clearly articulated rationale serves to motivate people to participate in the change process.

Our vision was to create excellence in supervision to ensure that our service users would meet the very best therapists we could be. Supervision is recognised as playing a key part in ensuring good practice and high-quality care (HCPC, 2022). Our aspiration was to have a professional reboot, to reenergise our teams to be excited, inspired and supported to participate in high quality professional supervision.

Our aims were to ensure:

- A clear and robust professional supervision structure
- Consistency of supervision practice
- Suitably trained staff to provide and receive supervision
- Effective systems of monitoring governance
- Assurance that staff were meeting professional standards for supervision

Kotter's Step 5: Enable action by removing barriers

Readers will notice that within this reflection I have missed Step 4 of Kotter's process. Kotter's 2018 model recognises that the steps in the process can be run concurrently and continuously, and on reflection, our project moved from Step 3 directly to Step 5. At this stage, Kotter gives examples of barriers such as inefficient processes, historical norms, and bureaucracy, outlining that by removing barriers, employees are provided with freedom to create change and make impact. The working group agreed it was essential to provide all staff with the opportunity to update their understanding of supervision, requiring an investment in training in supervision practices. Discussions took place considering attendance, cost, securing financial support, measuring the impact of the training against our aims, and sustainability and development of supervision to support future generations of therapists.

The group met for three meetings, over a six-month period, with delegated responsibilities and project time between meetings. We researched internal and external training opportunities and spoke to leaders in our professional field for guidance. There was no suitable training internally, but three external training providers were approached who were able to deliver suitable training packages, with various costs.

We wrote an options appraisal, which was shared with the senior leadership team, and were invited to present within a senior leadership meeting. We successfully secured a significant financial investment to provide external supervision training within the department. This was an amazing situation to be in and was a message of positivity towards our teams; the challenge then faced was to deliver on our vision.

The training plan

Every speech and language therapist and assistant was booked into the training sessions. Over one hundred staff (around 75% uptake) received a one-day foundation level training in supervision by an external professional supervision provider, over a two-week period.

Feedback from the course was positive, one speech and language therapist commenting that:

"I thought I was receiving supervision but now I realise that I haven't been".

Kotter's Step 4: Enlist a volunteer army

"Large-scale change can only occur when very significant numbers amass under a common opportunity and drive in the same direction" (Kotter, 2018, p19).

By providing training to such a large number of staff, we had, on reflection amassed our army of freshly trained and motivated therapists keen to engage in supervision practices. We were keen to ensure that any gains made through this investment in the current staff group could be sustained, considering new staff arriving, update training, maintenance of competencies. We agreed to identify supervision leaders in each geographical locality, the supervision "champions". Their role was to

- Coordinate supervision practices locally
- Respond to local supervision queries
- Form the ongoing working group
- Arrange and deliver rolling training for professional supervision
- Work alongside local operational managers to embed and maintain effective supervision practices
- Keep up to date with the evidence base and updated policies and guidelines relating to supervision

Staff who had expressed an interest in taking on the champions' role were then provided with a second day of supervision training. Around thirty staff attended this training.

Kotter's Step 6: Generating short term wins

Kotter describes the importance of short-term wins in the cycle of change. In our project, it was important for the team to maintain momentum, to demonstrate to both staff and senior leaders that the resource investment for training had been worthwhile, and to capitalise on the spirit of excitement and curiosity that the training had provided.

We arranged some immediate actions running concurrently with the training plan. An intranet site was set up to share resources, which included a library of documentation for supervision contracts, recording supervision sessions, and reflection documents. A database was set up, to enable the department to oversee who was receiving and providing supervision, to ensure equity of provision and access.

In the absence of clear professional and regulatory guidance at the time, an updated local supervision protocol was written. It outlined supervision practices including the roles and responsibilities (e.g., managers, supervision champions, and individual staff members); how the department would ensure all staff were appropriately trained; the time commitment from the organisation and from individual staff; how to select a supervisor; supervision contacts; supervision documentation and the information governance of this documentation; and how and when to access external supervision. This document was widely shared and stored on the supervision intranet for easy access.

A clear system of provision of managerial supervision (as defined by RCSLT, 2017) was employed across our organisation, using a standardised process, format and documentation. Within regular line management supervision, discussions took place supporting clinicians to engage in professional supervision.

Kotter's Step 7: Sustaining acceleration

The analogy used by Kotter (2018) at this stage of the change process is that of driving a car. By now, the change is well underway, and some quick wins have taken place. He encourages us not to take our foot off the accelerator, rather to push harder to use the quick wins as momentum to further fuel the change. There is recognition that resistance and complacency are never far away.

As I reflect, I notice that our project entered this phase. We were keen to maintain the momentum of the project, and to ensure that supervision practices were truly embedded in our everyday working lives. The original working group was expanded to embrace the newly trained supervision champions. I recall that the meetings were innovative, dynamic, and positive, with participants feeling energised and inspired to drive forward changes in professional supervision practices. There was discussion of how to share knowledge within the wider profession, via writing articles and blog posts, alongside planning how to run internal supervision courses and how to audit the impact of professional supervision practices on staff well-being, professional practice, and patient care.

The systems and processes were in place, training had taken place, and clinical and operational leaders maintained the supervision conversation within individual meetings, team meetings, and in corridor conversations. Within local teams, changes were being seen, more staff were coming forward requesting supervision, and the database of staff was growing to demonstrate an increase of supervision uptake. Optimistically, it seemed that supervision cultures and practices were changing. NHS England (2018, p.20) outline principles for achieving change and discuss the need for "energy of change" to mobilise and motivate change. At this time within our project, it seemed that our five energies of change (social, spiritual, psychological, physical and intellectual) were aligned.

Kotter's Step 8: Institute change

This phase of change is concerned with sustainability, the stage at which the new ways of working are woven firmly into the fabric of the organisational business. Kotter recognises that this stage can take many years, and that cultural changes take place far down the line of transformational change, and not at the beginning.

What happened next will not be an unusual story within health organisations. Shortly after the implementation of the new supervision structures in 2016, our organisation went through a period of restructure and reorganisation. The leadership changed, and the impetus and oversight of the supervision project was lost. Consequently, we did not reach the stage of institutionalising our cultural changes in supervision practices. The working group lay abandoned, with smaller, local teams being left to continue the work in newly formed structures. In retrospect, this hiatus in the project enabled an unforeseen and natural opportunity to consolidate our project aims within teams, but at the time there was a sense that all the excellent work that had taken place had been lost.

In 2017, the RCSLT published new information on supervision, which provided clarity on the issues our department had been grappling with, and as such, superseded the local supervision protocols. This latest information was widely shared with all SLT staff and service managers, but there were no further attempts to regain the momentum of the supervision project.

Where are we now?

Some eight years on from the outset of this project, supervision practices have been revisited by SLT teams. This has been prompted by an awareness by leadership teams that previously gained improvements in professional supervision practices were slipping; an increasing number of staff were not engaging in professional supervision or had not received supervision training. The new light shining from behind the clouds is a tangible energy within the team. A small, but different group of champions has reviewed the professional supervision practices, guidelines, and evidence base. This group consists of therapists new to the team, a senior leader, two of the original champions' group, all of whom have a passion for supervision. These therapists have attended a further external training course and meet on a regular basis to review emerging guidance, and lead on professional supervision practices. An internal supervision training package has been developed, and training is held, led by the supervision champions, three times a year for new staff and as refresher training as needed.

We have recently measured the impact of the supervision training on supervisees within the team, by conducting a review using the Manchester clinical supervision scale, MCSS-26© (Winstanley and White, 2011). This evaluation survey was distributed to all SLT staff, and the data was statistically analysed. Overall, the findings were positive, comparing favourably with those from other international studies using the MCSS-26 © tool. Eighty-five percent of respondents reported being moderately or very satisfied with the clinical supervision they receive. It has been valuable to gain this insight and assurance about this element of professional practice, and to validate the financial, intellectual and resource investment. The understanding of the true impact of supervision practices on patient care remains elusive, perhaps this is the next stage in the evolution of supervision research in SLT.

Reflections and sharing learning

Reflecting on this long journey through the change management model has enabled me to realise that we have come a long way. Unwittingly, we have moved through the stages of change outlined by John Kotter and have navigated the uncertain waters of the NHS. We have reached the point of evaluation and plan for further refinement. The volume of work that has taken place to build an operational infrastructure that supports robust supervision is considerable, but both professional and managerial supervision are now well-established constructs within the service.

At the outset of the project, I naively harboured a sense of optimism that changes in culture and practice would take place across clinical teams in a shorter timeframe after such a considerable resource investment. John Kotter's words encapsulate my learning from this experience that "Years of different kinds of experience are often needed to create lasting change" (2018, p. 30). In the fast-paced and under-resourced climate of the NHS, the timeframe of our project perhaps reflects the reality of leading change and implementing new models of practice whilst juggling multiple demands and priorities. Kotter argues that many change projects fail because victory is declared too early. This certainly rings true in my ears. I realise that within a large organisation, which has complicated infrastructures, diverse personnel, and multiple demands, that change takes time, and usually a lot more time than you initially anticipate. What the supervision journey for my organisation has exemplified is that you cannot plan for, nor account for internal and external influences on a project yet there can be value gained through facing these challenges.

Arguably, eight years ago, the timing may not have been optimal for the delivery of regular internal professional supervision training. How can we account for the fact that the team has had only recent success in the realisation of the vision of whole staff groups having regular support for professional supervision and training? Timeliness, and readiness for change seem critical; perhaps the small seeds sewn in the initial supervision training needed time to germinate to enable a critical mass of therapists to embrace professional supervision and realise the change.

Project learning for readers' consideration

1. Options Appraisals and Project plans

Consider options for change at the outset by using options appraisal methodology and construct a clear project plan. This process enables the development of a realistic understanding of the problem, creating a clear vision, the scale, costs, and time requirement to deliver the implementation plan. (e.g., NHS Improving Quality 2014; NHS England (2018), The Health Foundation, 2021). Project management systems provide tools for close and effective monitoring of a project, enabling clear and regular review of the project deliverables (e.g. PRINCE2, Bennett, 2017).

Within the context of NHS services, performance indicators are largely driven by quantitative data, such as referral to treatment times, caseload figures, and efficient appointment bookings. Measurement of a project implementing supervision practices is an inherently indirect professional activity, so that in this context, measurements of engagement with supervision within the service (quantitative) alongside qualitative data capturing the granularity of the personal experience and impact to both clients and staff would be useful measurements to consider from the project outset.

2. Measurement of change

Consider implementing a robust and detailed audit tool from the outset, to enable baseline as well as outcome measures. In our project, an online anonymous baseline questionnaire could have been used at the outset, alongside staff focus groups, to gain a wider baseline measure using both qualitative and quantitative data. James Harrington succinctly underlines this:

"Measurement is the first step that leads to control and eventually to improvement. If you can't measure something, you can't understand it. If you can't understand it, you can't control it. If you can't control it, you can't improve it." (NHS Quality Improvement, 2014, p31).

3. Consider organisational climate

Undertaking an analysis of influencing variables within the organisation at the commencement of the project may be beneficial, such as the use of a PESTLE analysis (Pestle Analysis 2021). Identification of political, economic, sociological, technological, legal and environmental factors which are influencing the current state, enables potential barriers to be anticipated and managed.

4. Create an effective team

Consider key people to lead professional supervision practices. Having a team of therapists who were curious, open minded, passionate about supervision, and had an energy to change practice and bring people "on board" was critical in influencing change. Having a spread of staff across the career profiles enables a wider perspective and supports successful dissemination and engagement across teams. This also creates opportunities for growth and leadership development of junior staff.

Keeping the project group small but representative enables meetings to be set up easily, to keep to agendas and timescales, to share ownership of the project and its aims. Having a member of the senior leadership team on the working group supports effective communication between the working group and the management team.

In the pressured world of clinical practice, too often improvement projects are squeezed into time slots in diaries, or rescheduled due to patient demand, or reliant on the goodwill of professionals to complete work within their own time. Critical to consider is the additional time requirement for the supervision champions to participate in meetings, develop and run the internal training package. This responsibility and time commitment was reflected in individual job plans.

5. Seek support from external agencies

Consider who your 'critical friends' are and how they can benefit your project. For us, commissioning an external training provider gave validity and credibility to the information imparted, and supported the project team through the journey.

6. Consider sustainability

Keep the vision in mind and carry it into the future with regular nurturing. Within a fast-paced, ever-changing environment, clinicians are bombarded with the next change in practice, and focus is taken away from the achievements already made. Rather like the need to nurture a sapling for it to become a tree, there is need for constant attention towards newly embedded practices to maintain growth and development.

7. Practice Self Care

Leading change is complex, and the challenges cannot be underestimated within the vastness and complexity of health environments. Consideration should be given to ensuring support is available to the project team, through project coaches, and robust supervision structures. Formal reflective sessions, such as Action Learning, have been valuable (NHS England, 2015). I found that my own professional supervision was critical. I used this safe, confidential space to explore the project challenges, and to celebrate successes, share my frustrations and "check in" whether my perceptions and intuition were sound.

Concluding thoughts

After eight years, I am confident that our supervision culture and practices have developed positively and feel assured of this through the recent supervision evaluation findings, and practices within the service. Through the sometimes slow and deliberate chiselling away of the rocks of outdated professional practice, we are now uncovering the shining crystals of supervision excellence within our teams, the success of which can be attributed to the passion and commitment of the supervision champions and the therapists who participate in regular professional and managerial supervision. I hope that by reflecting on the highs and lows of our journey, using Kotter's 8 step model, other organisations will be inspired, motivated, and prepared to embed a culture of robust supervision practices within their teams.

Note

1 RCSLT (2017) uses the terms Professional Supervision and Managerial Supervision. Prior to that, Clinical supervision was the term most identified within SLT, differentiating it from managerial supervision. Throughout this chapter, professional

supervision will be the term used when describing a supervision agreement outside of the line management structure, and supervision as the overarching term for both managerial and professional supervision.

References

AWSLTMC All Wales Speech and Language Therapy Managers Committee (2008) *Clinical Supervision Guidelines.* Unpublished.

Bennett, N. A. (2017) *Managing Successful Projects with Prince2,* 6th edition UK: TSO.

HCPC (2016) *Standards of Proficiency – Speech and Language Therapists.* London: HCPC. Viewed 30 August 2022 at www.hcpc-uk.org/standards/standards-of-proficiency/speech-and-language-therapists/

HCPC (2022) *What is supervision?* London: HCPC. Viewed 30 August 2022 at www.hcpc-uk.org/standards/meeting-our-standards/supervision-leadership-and-culture/supervision/what-is-supervision/

Kotter, J. (2018) *8 Steps to Accelerate Change in your Organisation.* Boston: Kotter. Viewed 30 Aug 2022 at www.kotterinc.com

Kotter, J. (1996) *Leading Change.* Boston USA: Harvard Business School Press.

NHS England (2015) *NHS Improving Quality Learning Handbook: Action Learning Sets.* NHS England. Viewed 6 September 2022 at www.england.nhs.uk

NHS England (2018) *The Change Model Guide.* England: NHS England. Viewed 30 August 2022 at www.england.nhs.uk/publication/the-change-model-guide/

NHS Improving Quality (2014) *First Steps Towards Quality Improvement: A Simple Guide to Improving Services.* Viewed 6 July 2024 at www.england.nhs.uk/improvement-hub/wp-content/uploads/sites/44/2011/06/service_improvement_guide_2014.pdf

Pestle (2021) *What is a PESTLE Analysis? An important Business analysis tool* Viewed 30 August 2022 at https://pestleanalysis.com/pestel-model/

RCSLT (2012) *Supervision Guidelines for Speech and Language Therapists.* London: RCSLT.

RCSLT (2017) *Information on Supervision.* London: RCSLT.

The Health Foundation (2021) *Quality improvement made simple. What everyone should know about health care quality improvement.* Viewed 6 July 2024 at reader.health.org.uk/qi-made-simple-2021

Winstanley, J. and White E. (2011) The MCSS-26©: revision of The Manchester Clinical Supervision Scale© using the Rasch Measurement Model. *Journal of Nursing Measurement,* 19:3, pp160–178

6 The Alchemy of Group Supervision

Penny Farrell, Jennifer Roche, Edel O'Dea and Lauren Tyson (née Wright)

We are a group of speech and language therapists (SLTs) working across Ireland and the United Kingdom. Our roles are diverse and span the independent, publicly funded, and voluntary sector, delivering interventions for children and adults who stammer. We work in education, advocacy and strategic planning. Most of us have never met in person.

Our online supervision group formed in September 2020 around our common interest in working with people who stammer from the perspective of the neurodiversity paradigm and critical disability theory (Campbell, Constantino & Simpson, 2019; Constantino, Campbell & Simpson, 2022). In this chapter, we describe our experience of facilitated group supervision and how it creates an essential, dynamic and nurturing space for reflective practice, professional wellbeing and personal flourishing as we strive to embrace a neurodiversity-affirming approach to stammering (Constantino, 2018; Gerlach-Houck & Constantino, 2022; Constantino, 2023).

We appreciate that our readers will bring their own experiences, assumptions, perspectives and expectations about group supervision and stammering as they engage with this chapter. It is our hope we might surprise our readers with the myriad benefits of our group and encourage them to seek a similar opportunity.

We wish to clarify that the facilitated group supervision outlined in this chapter is not intended to replace traditional forms of professional supervision. Instead, we propose external facilitated group supervision can be a complementary experience.

DOI: 10.4324/9781003301141-6

Our shared perspective on stammering

Our philosophical approach to stammering is not universally shared by clients or colleagues working in this specialist field. While it is increasingly recognised as valid (St. Pierre, 2012; Constantino, Campbell & Simpson, 2022), some of our readers may not have encountered this perspective of stammering.

As a group of SLTs, we continue to travel on a journey transitioning from a predominantly medicalised deficit-based definition and model of stammering therapy towards a philosophy and practice that honours verbal diversity. We actively seek to learn and reflect on the complex, multi-faceted and unique experiences of people who stammer.

We aspire to facilitate insights and provide support so clients can make sense of their story within a societal context, make informed choices and explore how to dismantle barriers to communicating confidently, with increased spontaneity and joy in their identity as people who stammer. Alongside navigating an unpredictable pattern to the flow of speech, there can be an emotional response and reactivity to stammering. This can be borne out of and compounded by negative bias and ableist assumptions. This may trigger or amplify internalised stigma, trauma, physical struggle and concealment of stammering.

We see our role as collaborators, working in partnership with the stammering community and allies, in advocating for a greater understanding and acceptance of stammering as a valid way of speaking. We want to create a culture where, for instance, young children who stammer receive support to prevent the adverse impact of ableist assumptions on their self-esteem and identity as effective communicators, whether their stammer remains present as they grow or not.

Adapting our practice to honour our shared philosophy and aspirations is akin to rebuilding a ship at sea. We must navigate a legacy of ableist therapy practices and unhelpful societal assumptions about stammering, which surround us as therapists and our clients. It is a delicate task requiring openness to, and acceptance of, therapist uncertainty and treading carefully lest the ship capsizes. Our supervision group is a dedicated space where we can navigate this voyage in solidarity. There is an alchemy at work in this open, authentic and collaborative group encounter.

This chapter presents an overview of our group as we describe and analyse the supervision process. We draw parallels with growing creativity, moving beyond boundaries as a group, developing advancing practice and the ripple effect to personal and professional life. We illustrate the roles of presenter, listener and facilitator and invoke reflections on skill development and personal growth.

The format of our supervision group

Our group was created following a message on social media from our facilitator. It was an invitation to create a new supervision group to support the integration of critical disability theory into practice in relation to stammering. We met for an initial no-obligation exploratory session where we discussed what we would like from this opportunity and we explored the possibility of drawing on action learning set principles to bring structure to the encounter.

Action Learning (McGill & Beaty, 2001) is based on the principle that individuals achieve most of their knowledge through practical experience. Traditionally, it brings together 6–8 individuals in a 'set' who are neither direct colleagues nor in line management relationships, thereby allowing more freedom to express vulnerability and uncertainty.

Our group agreed to commit to meeting once a month for two hours. It draws on, rather than strictly complies with, action learning principles. The description that follows reflects the verbal agreement between us regarding the format of the group. We reflect on the aspects of our unique group process which we have found helpful, and may be of benefit to the reader.

Checking in

At the start of each supervision meeting, we check in by acknowledging where we are with the hubris of life. We share 'trauma, trivia or joy' (McGill & Beaty, 2001: 109) as we adjust from our private space to the meeting. In doing so, we allow these things to rest so we can focus on the forthcoming session and be fully present with a clearer mind. This is helpful in an online meeting, when there is no transition or travel time beforehand. Checking in and acknowledging our common humanity, creates an atmosphere of trust, openness and solidarity from the outset which holds true for the remainder of the session.

Bidding

Next, there is a bidding process to agree on who will present and share a specific issue, concern or dilemma. Group members may offer a scenario, practice issue or discussion point for consideration. The group decides by consensus on two bids to explore across the two-hour session and the first presenter then holds the floor.

Presenting and exploring the issue

The presenters are given uninterrupted time to reflect and verbalise spontaneously, teasing out all the strands of the issue they are grappling with. To create a safe space and become attentive and mindful listeners, we agree to not take written notes during the session.

After the presentation process, listeners are invited to ask questions for clarification, which come from a place of genuine naivety to the situation. These questions are not judgemental, loaded or advisory. The listeners are the beneficiaries of the first round of questions as the questions they ask seek clarity to their understanding of the situation. Sometimes, as a presenter, these questions prompt us to wonder why we had not revealed that information within our initial description and what that means about how we have approached the problem. Other times we are unable to answer, giving us another piece of the puzzle to try to understand.

The presenter is at the heart of the second round of questions. Questioning now invites the presenter to reflect more deeply on the situation and expand their understanding of it. Stimulating and energising questioning leads to deeper self-examination as a presenter, guiding us to tap into our own ideology and values, thereby creating a space to develop a fresh viewpoint. Exploring these levels of understanding and exposing gaps or contradictions can feel unsettling. However, the group responds with encouragement and respect, possibly because we empathise with the profound insight that we are each experiencing. Feeling this mutual enjoyment of learning gives us the freedom to bring problems that make the most difference to our professional development and clinical practice.

Following the exploration of the problem, the group takes turns to share their reflections and observations with the presenter. These may relate to body sensations, thoughts, or feelings, resonating personal or professional experiences or what informed or challenged the questioning process.

Rounding off the process this way offers more fresh perspectives, enriching their issue further. We can appreciate we are not alone, and our issues receive empathy and are not a solitary concern.

Finally comes the time for the presenter to speak from their position, responding with concluding reflections and insights that have been precipitated by the full circle of the process.

Reflections on the process

As our group holds shared values about stammering, the experience of being a listener and presenter is equally beneficial. Listening is energising. Assumptions such as 'this might not be relevant for me' and 'this is someone else's learning opportunity', dissolved when we realised the powerful gains of the listener role. Listening grants insights into other's work lives, practice, what we are grappling with and the views we hold.

Our role as listener is not to look directly for answers to offer the presenter, but rather to ask questions that expand their perspective of the situation. Finding a 'truth' is not the objective and so answers are not required from the listeners. As therapists, our clients and colleagues often view us as experts, as people who will talk from our viewpoint, identify solutions and fix their problems, and sometimes we adopt this role. In the supervision group we resist this urge and cultivate our skills to keep the focus on the presenter, stay in their frame of reference and hold our questions in mind until the speaker has finished. In this way, the listeners are central to the presenter's enquiry process.

Being a listener can be difficult, especially as the process involves not taking written notes. How do we remember what is said and not miss useful segments of knowledge? We have learned to trust the process of listening wholly and going with the flow of thoughts and questions. The beauty of the group format and our dynamic is that things do not need to be perfect. We can be raw and honest with each other. Listening to understand keeps us grounded in the here and now. Our shared vulnerability is a tonic. Our minds are not distracted by how others might perceive us. We can be truly open about our learning needs without trying to impress one another and appear all-knowing.

The process requires courage and authenticity. Reflecting openly about our experiences, strengths and vulnerabilities as therapists was initially challenging for us all and the gains have been myriad. By allowing our professional peers to share dilemmas and aspirations at a deeper level, to empathise and imagine within the group, there has been 'sparking' of both individual and collective thinking and new insights have emerged.

Presenters have sometimes come with situations and problems that are completely different to those which occur in other group members' practice, yet still, we have found commonality and relevance. As professionally we often work in isolation, it is a privilege to be around like-minded therapists. It feels like we are travelling together in one car, sharing a love for the same genre of music, and we are bringing along new tracks we may or may not have heard of before. The whole process feels open and honest, rich and intimate.

As therapists, bringing these qualities into our own clinical practice has had a positive impact for the people we work with. We can give others our full attention, trusting ourselves to be present and respond congruently. By being fully present we can listen deeply and that alone can be extremely powerful.

The empowering dynamic of facilitated group supervision

Our facilitator

Our supervision sessions differ from non-facilitated peer supervision. We are guided by our facilitator, who is a professional colleague, as she accompanies us along a process that trusts in the dynamic of a group encounter. We feel privileged that our facilitator brings a unique mix of wisdom and experience to this pivotal role, as a speech and language therapist, supervisor, person-centred counsellor, educator and activist with a deep understanding of critical disability theory and its importance in informing our role in working with people who stammer. This combination undoubtedly crafted a warm, compassionate, inviting, empathetic, and safe space for a group of people who had never met before.

When our group first formed, we initially benefited from our facilitator's guidance to ensure we kept within the intention of each stage as we moved through the enquiry process from bidding to presenting, from asking questions to reflecting. She supported us to be present for each other, to listen, to seek understanding, enquire, and share reflections and observations in turn. She kept time, both holding space and moving us on through the process when needed so that each stage was honoured as intended and our attention absorbed in the content of the group. She distilled the shared wisdom and themes that emerged from the group and helped create clarity around our shared dilemmas.

There is much to admire in how our facilitator empowers us all to feel confident, be vulnerable, be curious and take our time. She has a wonderful ability to reflect back what we are thinking in a way we may not be able to articulate ourselves. As the group has progressed and we have become more familiar and confident with the process, there has been a shift in the group power dynamic towards less support from the facilitator and a more equal distribution of agency with our increasing experience and confidence.

Readers who would like to adopt this format would benefit from a facilitator who can promote, validate and develop these generative skills in the group participants.

Acknowledging vulnerability and nurturing new learning

For some of us, our prior supervision was led by a manager and was connected to our personal learning plans and learning measures. Earlier in our careers, formats of supervision often had a predefined structure and outcome, which left us feeling a lack of ownership over the agenda and process of learning. Perhaps there was also a subconscious inclination to hold back for self-protection, hindering the potential for genuine learning and growth.

Prior peer-to-peer group supervision with our own departmental colleagues sometimes involved unclear boundaries or unfacilitated formats. To ensure everyone had their turn, issues felt hurriedly addressed and therefore leaned heavily towards advice-giving. Whilst valuable and supportive, there was not enough time to fully explore an issue and there was an air of needing to prove oneself to demonstrate our own expertise and competence to our colleagues.

By contrast, navigating our own session agenda in our facilitated group has been a novel experience for some of us. The freedom of entering a session with a blank canvas and collaboratively crafting a vibrant masterpiece is refreshing.

The absence of colleague relationships in our group has cultivated an environment where openness and vulnerability are welcomed without worrying about judgement, appearing uninformed or lacking in expertise.

With the support of the facilitator, we work safely outside our comfort zones, allow ourselves to be open and to speak about and to our vulnerabilities. This has needed trust in the process and each other. Stepping outside of our comfort zone has stretched us 'just enough' and created a safe space that facilitated deeper reflections, personal and professional learning and growth that we have rarely experienced in other supervision formats. In our group we are enquiring and creative therapists who hold and explore uncertainty with increasing confidence. Our identity as therapists has strengthened and the shared wisdom and experience of our supervisor and peers has been internalised.

Edel reflects on the power of the group dynamic from a personal perspective. It brought up a memory for her of attending several visual art classes. Individual students would face their easels while the expert, an accomplished artist, demonstrated techniques, circulated around the studio, made suggestions and often intervened directly to ensure each student had a respectable finished piece of art. There was minimal interaction between students apart from trivial chat and exchange of compliments. By contrast, Edel experienced a more dynamic and interactive group learning experience in an advanced fine art course. Tutors rarely demonstrated their own technical and creative skills, instead, the group benefited from their facilitation skills. The tutor brought a diverse group of students along a collaborative journey of uncertainty, enquiry and experimental practice. Students took turns to present their work, describing the theme they were exploring and narrating their creative process. They initially felt vulnerable in their roles of presenter, observer and listener, in case they were exposed as an 'imposter' as their identities as artists were fragile. However, the impact on creativity was exponential. Instead of focusing in a blinkered way on their individual project, students engaged in the creative process of the entire group. They continuously moved outside the boundaries they might have set for themselves, becoming more adventurous and confident in their identity as artists. The synergy of the group dynamic was empowering, and students drew on that energy and internalised wisdom to inspire and motivate themselves when initiating fine art projects in solitude at home. The experience of our supervision group has had a similar generative dynamic.

Edel reflects that, as a therapist with decades of experience, she initially felt anxious about exposing her inadequacies or ableist blind spots about stammering when she stepped into the presenter or listener roles during this group process. The ongoing support of our facilitator alongside growing familiarity with the roles of presenter and listener were aided by the burgeoning trust with the other group members. Edel noticed that over time the internal voice popping up with the word 'imposter' faded and was replaced with a voice that celebrated the strength of sharing uncertainty. The sessions offer a valuable opportunity for honest, collaborative enquiry.

The group facilitation style, combined with being facilitated to explore practice through the lens of critical disability theory, is an opportunity for growth as a therapist and human being. Supporting a minority view against the established view through group supervision has led to a wider awareness of the range of issues and biases that need to be challenged.

Benefits that extend beyond enhanced clinical skills

On reflection, it is unlikely many of us would have connected in our day-to-day clinical practices, and even if we had, we would not be holding the connection and bond cemented from our shared group supervision. Over time, our understanding and insight into each other's lives has deepened, and whilst this remains professional, it feels like we see each other in our true and authentic forms, as whole human beings, rather than being defined by our job titles. Despite being in two different countries and working across completely different healthcare sectors, there is a strong feeling of community and camaraderie between us.

Integration into clinical practice

Penny and Lauren reflect on this from personal perspectives.

Penny writes: My experience of learning about disability theory and how to embody this as a therapist has been more akin to Penrose stairs (Penrose & Penrose, 1958) than a linear learning curve. Just as I come to a clear understanding of my values and how I can align these with my role as a therapist, I turn the corner and become aware of more stairs to climb. Were it not for the group, I suspect I would be sitting somewhere further down the steps, feeling unsure of my direction or how to move forwards on this journey. There is a sincerity and vulnerability in the group process that has clarified my thoughts and emboldened me to embrace a new paradigm. We all need our champions when we venture somewhere new, and this group has done just that. Through the vulnerability of sharing so openly in our supervision group, I better appreciate the value of learning as a process, not an outcome.

Lauren continues: While writing this, I have chosen to embrace spontaneity and see where my thoughts lead. Typically, I would consult my written notes and anticipate my responses. Engaging in this unscripted process is novel for me. I used to prioritise session plans, equating success with completing every aspect. I realise a successful therapy session is not confined by predetermined boundaries, instead, it thrives when tailored to meet the individual where they are, addressing what they wish to discuss and what would be most beneficial for them.

I also discovered the importance of challenging assumptions I would have previously accepted without scrutiny. My perspective has evolved and I now approach everything with a different lens, fostering a habit of increased questioning. Our group has empowered me to experiment with new approaches in my practice, ranging from altering assessment questions to establishing an outdoor therapy group for children who stammer.

Integration into professional supervision

Penny reflects on her previous experience of professional supervision compared to group supervision drawing on action learning principles.

As a student in the late 90s, I was introduced to Peyton's Learning Cycle (Peyton, 1998) which hypothesises four stages of learning in clinical education:

1. Unconscious incompetence
2. Conscious incompetence
3. Conscious competence
4. Unconscious competence

Using this model, I realise that the way I participated in much of my previous supervision was to prove to myself and my peers that I was in stage three of conscious competence. I felt compelled to show what I knew, how I knew it and how I applied my knowledge. Supervision often felt like a test I had to pass rather than a learning experience. I was afraid of asking 'silly' questions or being truly open about challenges I faced, in case they led to criticism or negative judgement. The format I experience in this supervision group allows me to be more authentic, enabling me to explore the multi-faceted layers of the issue without concern for how I may be perceived. This is very freeing. The more I openly explored and allowed my vulnerabilities to be aired, with support and constructive reflections, confidence in myself began to grow. Many times, I felt reassured I could cycle through various stages and resolve my queries through the group 'think-tank'. This gave me further reassurance and confidence that I did have the knowledge and skills. I benefit from the allocated time and supportive space to think it through. The process is reciprocal as I observe my peers go through a similar process arising from my reflections and feedback for them. This helps me feel more empowered about supporting group members without giving prescriptive advice. By pooling my thoughts with the rest of the group, we generate a medley of shared insights and learning.

Bringing it all together

Here, we individually reflect on what the group supervision process has given us and conclude the chapter with our shared thoughts.

Jen writes: Facilitated group supervision has been a profound experience for me. Having a clear focus and a repeated structure is comforting. I know what to expect and still each session is unique and inspiring. Learning alongside people from a range of different contexts, with a diversity of experiences who are all connected by a shared clinical specialism, being heard with pure interest and respect, being questioned to foster my new insights, and hearing how my experience resonates to theirs is a privilege. Working through one, defined and distinct problem helps me to make headway with that, but also brings into relief new possibilities and illuminates ideas I had not been cognisant of before; solving problems before I had labelled them as such. The effect is immense.

I feel blessed to be part of a group whose professional roles include being a listener. I have learned to listen with greater attentiveness to really understand, to encourage speakers to cultivate their insights through my own silence and to ask questions which invite the speaker to examine their situation more deeply.

In my clinical work, more therapy groups are available with more space to explore nuanced themes which are brought by the group itself. I find myself increasingly responding to the needs of the group as they arise. The groups are taking more ownership of the routes we take on these journeys. The same is true of my practice as a professional supervisor.

Penny adds: The alchemy of our group conversations has sparked new understandings and increased confidence for me. The group has offered me a protected space to examine issues or challenges with curiosity and openness. Sometimes learning is only visible retrospectively. I look back and see how things have changed in what I do, how I do it and why. In a similar way to my thoughts about stammering pride, there is not a final definitive end point. It is a journey, not a destination and it is an honour to journey with my fellow travel companions.

Edel continues: As a therapist I found myself contemplating the possible end to a long career during a pandemic that radically changed how we functioned in our personal and professional lives. Participating in an online facilitated supervision group with therapists engaging with critical disability theory has reinvigorated the joy in my identity as a speech and language therapist. I have been able to acknowledge with honesty just how challenged and vulnerable I can feel at times by the implicit expectations created by my professional title alone. The attentive listening, gentle inquiry and thoughtful reflection and wisdom that we share under the guidance of our facilitator allows me to tease out the myriad strands of a dilemma and view any scenario with fresh clarity. Through the group, I have developed an expanded concept of my role that incorporates advocacy and education. I realise I am not ready to relinquish the challenges and joys of being a therapist and I feel empowered instead to journey onwards.

The synergy of our group process is a catalyst for both personal and professional growth, confidence and flourishing; a process worth seeking in other spheres of my life. As I reflect on my experience, I can see how vital it is for SLT students and practising therapists who choose this brave career to experience a sense of being held and nurtured in a safe space as they navigate the ethical dilemmas and uncertainties that are a part of professional growth.

Lauren adds: Being around therapists grappling with evolving perspectives on stammering has been important to me. The group has played a crucial role in gaining clarity on my values and beliefs, revealing I do not have to adhere to an 'all or nothing' approach. I have learned to embrace fluidity and allow myself to shift and adapt as needed. This flexibility has involved navigating new understandings and challenging outdated beliefs that no longer resonate with me. The group provides a platform to collaboratively navigate these transitions with others, fostering the exchange of diverse perspectives and experiences that enrich our collective exploration. I learned the paramount importance of professional supervision. It is not a practice to casually engage with, it is indispensable and requires regular commitment.

Concluding thoughts

Alchemy serves as a powerful metaphor for the transformative journey experienced within our supervision group. Individually the elements of this group supervision may not seem to be much, but once combined, they enable a magical, profound experience for all that has numerous and unexpected benefits.

We all agree the number of personal and professional gains from our sessions have transcended our expectations. We have faced challenges ranging from being honest and vulnerable, talking from raw and unedited points of view, to grappling with the complexities of ableism, stigma and language itself. We have unravelled complex thoughts and feelings, even when we could not fully articulate what these were. We have been deeply listened to, valued and respected. Ideas have been sparked with new and fresh perspectives. Boundaries have shifted, insights gained, confidence levels increased. We have expanded our clinical practices and beyond, benefitting the clients we serve and the organisations we work for. We have sat with discomfort, celebrated successes and drawn upon reflections with curious minds. We have embraced the process and experience of shared learning. We have evolved into our true authentic selves without fear of repercussions or judgements. We have developed genuine connections and we continue to champion and cheer each other on.

We hope our readers will be inspired by our story and perhaps be tempted or curious to try out this form of facilitated group supervision in parallel with other professional supervision formats.

References

Campbell, P., Constantino, C. and Simpson, S. (2019) *Stammering Pride and Prejudice: Difference Not Defect.* J & R Press.

Constantino, C. (2018) What can stutterers learn from the neurodiversity movement? *Seminars in Speech and Language,* 39(4), 382–396. https://doi.org/10.1055/s-0038-1667166

Constantino, C., Campbell, P. and Simpson, S. (2022) Stuttering and the social model. *Journal of Communication Disorders*, 96, 106200. https://doi.org/10.1016/j.jcomdis.2022.106200

Constantino, C. (2023) Fostering positive stuttering identities using stutter-affirming therapy. *Language, Speech and Hearing Services in Schools*, 54, 42–62. https://doi.org/10.1044/2022_LSHSS-22-00038

Gerlach-Houck, H. and Constantino, C. (2022) Interrupting ableism in stuttering therapy and research: Practical suggestions. *Perspectives of the ASHA Special Interest Groups*, 1–18. https://doi.org/10.1044/2021_PERSP-21-00109

McGill, I. & Beaty, L. (2001) *Action Learning: A Guide for Professional, Management & Educational Development*, 2nd edn. London: Routledge.

Penrose, L. S. and Penrose, R. (1958) Impossible objects: A special type of visual illusion, *British Journal of Psychology*, 49(1), 31–33. https://doi.org/10.1111/j.2044-8295.1958.tb00634.x

Peyton J. (1998) The Learning Cycle. In Peyton J., *Teaching and Learning in Medical Practice*. Manticore Europe Limited, 13–19.

St Pierre, J. (2012) The construction of the disabled speaker: Locating stuttering in disability studies. *Canadian Journal of Disability Studies*, 1(3). https://doi.org/10.15353/cjds.v1i3.54

7

A Life Jacket in Stormy Seas

Supervision for Speech and Language Therapists Working with Young People Who Have Mental Health Challenges

Melanie Cross

My professional journey started in the UK National Health Service (NHS) where I worked in community clinics, a child development centre and a language unit. I was given the key to the clinic, a brief orientation and left to get on with it and I think this helped me develop self-efficacy as a clinician. For many years, I had no professional supervision, so I really valued lunch with colleagues and Clinical Excellence Network meetings, where we provided each other with emotional and professional support. When I had children, it was hard to find flexible working opportunities, consequently, I began freelance work. Initially, I worked for a non-profit foster care organisation, then I added paid part-time work for a charity and a university and voluntary work for the Royal College of Speech and Language Therapists (RCSLT). I hugely enjoyed the cross fertilisation of theory, practice and influencing.

Carving out a role as initially the only speech and language therapist (SLT) in an expanding fostering organisation, I took on managerial responsibilities. I was busy, juggling life and work, learning a lot and mostly disregarding the negative effects it had on me. There were days when I felt sick before work and had nightmares about what had happened to the young people I worked with. It made me hug my children more and work harder. My professional supervision needs were ignored, the organisation saw it as

DOI: 10.4324/9781003301141-7

my responsibility as I was self-employed. I could not find any speech and language therapists in the same sort of role who could support me and I did not think I needed or could access the sort of supervision psychotherapy colleagues received.

I began to understand the value of professional supervision through my training as a Video Interaction Guider (VIG) and supervisor (AVIG, 2023). I was supported by skilled supervisors to reflect on videos of my interactions with clients and supervisees. I also began to supervise others, which prompted me to learn more about supervision. Eventually I began to receive professional supervision from an SLT, which helped me recognise that professional supervision is not an optional luxury, but crucial to effective work and life!

This chapter makes a case for the professional supervision I wish I had had as I struggled to understand unfamiliar organisations, complex young people, and why building therapeutic relationships could be so tricky when young people have mental health challenges. It is exciting that working in mental health is an emerging field for SLTs, but there are also risks to our professionalism and our own mental health, which supervision can help mitigate. I hope this chapter helps readers recognise what good professional supervision for SLTs in mental health settings looks like and empowers them to get the sort of 'life jacket' they need.

The challenges of working in mental health settings

My experiences and those of my supervisees have helped me identify recurrent themes that can arise in various mental health settings including the NHS, Social Emotional and Mental Health (SEMH) schools, social care and independent organisations. I will focus on four areas which often come up in supervision:

- Emotional challenges
- Traumatic environments
- Unfamiliar work cultures – uncharted waters
- How do SLTs fit into existing supervision systems?

Emotional challenges

I have vivid memories of my first days at an SEMH school. It was fascinating and terrifying in equal measure. I had never seen such levels of distress in young people or adults expressing limitless care and empathy. There were amazing people, foster carers, families, education staff, various 'therapists', social workers, admin staff etc., and endearing young people, some of whom behaved in frightening ways at times. I was puzzled by the cynicism I witnessed too, including the use of 'restraints' which I found unsettling and at odds with attempts to understand the causes of young people's emotional dysregulation.

Other SLTs I have spoken to experience similar strong feelings when working with young people who have mental health challenges. There is also rage about inequality, the lack of recognition of speech language and communication needs (SLCN) and the paucity of services for those who experience them as well as the frequent changes of foster placement and school. In addition to this, there is 'emotional contagion' where young peoples' negative emotions can be passed on to people around them. The practitioner might not know this has happened until they act in an unexpected way, such as crying in a meeting. Ideally, professional supervision offers a space where SLTs are comfortable to explore the emotional challenges they encounter with a supervisor who is familiar with these issues and skilful in supporting them. I will discuss how this can be facilitated in more detail in the second section of this chapter.

Traumatic environments

In my experience, supporting young people with mental health challenges can be especially difficult when the young people or the practitioner bring a history of unresolved emotional trauma. This is shockingly common. One study found that almost 66% of a large nationally representative sample of young people had been exposed to more than one traumatic event, 30% had been exposed to five or more and 10% had experienced eleven or more (Turner et al., 2010). Many young people in mental health settings have experienced complex trauma involving multiple events with interpersonal threats (UK Trauma Council, no date). This means that SLTs are very likely to work with young people who have experienced trauma, as well as working alongside colleagues, or with supervisors, or supervisees who have direct experience of trauma.

Research suggests that those who have experienced childhood trauma often have elevated levels of empathy (Greenberg et al., 2018), and this may contribute to the motivation for working in this field. I have often observed SLTs describe a young person's outrageous behaviour with a smile on their face. This shows a wonderful capacity to 'see behind the behaviour', however, issues can arise when SLTs over-empathise, or over-identify with young people to the detriment of their own self-care.

Even if practitioners have no trauma history, working with young people who have mental health challenges, especially those who have experienced abuse and neglect, can be traumatising. Personally, stories about young people having to eat out of bins or being groomed by paedophile rings are hard to forget. Reading client records or learning about attachment and trauma can also spark insights which challenge assumptions and can be disconcerting. For example, there might be a recognition of unmet attachment needs, or a reappraisal of childhood experiences as traumatic.

Those who are empathic or who have unresolved trauma experiences may be particularly susceptible to secondary trauma. Research indicates this is common in the helping professions (Bridger et al., 2020), but not always recognised, including in speech and language therapy. In my experience, this work can be exhausting, leading to anxiety and feelings of helplessness, manifesting in all sorts of splits throughout an organisation which can ultimately be dangerous. Professional supervision is vital to being able to work effectively in traumatic environments, not least in recognising whether or when practitioners need more specialist psychological support.

Unfamiliar work cultures – uncharted waters

I notice that, as SLTs have begun to work in unfamiliar work cultures, they encounter different ideas about professionalism including confidentiality, self-disclosure, stress management and work life balance. Settings might prioritise systems, processes or relationships. The ethos might be 'sink or swim' or be emotionally available to the young people until overwhelmed and sometimes they mirror the chaos in the young people's lives.

I have frequently observed different perspectives on young people's strengths and 'needs'. SLTs challenge the established view by arguing that SLCN is an important and overlooked factor and by advocating for appropriate services. They may have to explain their role and what they can contribute, repeatedly. I have found that many young people with SEMH issues have complex needs, so working alongside them, their families and colleagues in order to support them is important. However, SLTs may not be included in the relevant meetings or processes, so professional supervision is often used to explore ways to facilitate collaboration.

In my opinion, SLTs in emerging roles have to balance their unique contribution with the requirements of the setting. They need to make sure they are not being pushed into ways of working that do not feel in the best interests of young people, or themselves. For example, questions that often arise in the professional supervision I offer include:

- Whose role is it to decide when and how SLTs assess and intervene?
- Who is in control of timetables/appointments and is that acceptable?
- Who evaluates what SLTs do and how?
- Should SLTs take part in physical interventions?

In my experience, SLTs can find themselves working in a culture that does not routinely offer or receive professional supervision. I have noticed that SLTs working in contexts where supervision is not offered or effective can become magnets for stressed colleagues who need to offload, perhaps because they are trained listeners. Consequently, SLTs must consider the impact this might have on them, and what to do with the difficult emotions it can provoke. Similarly, I think SLTs have to be careful about who they share their anxieties with, especially where there is no transparency about confidentiality within the organisation. For example, one SLT I know expressed a concern about how a young person was treated in what she thought was a confidential meeting, but her comments were repeated to the practitioner involved. This highlights the importance of independent, confidential supervision when reflecting on personal and organisational boundaries.

How do SLTs fit into existing supervision systems?

SLTs might think 'any port in a storm' when offered professional supervision in unfamiliar work environments, but I have seen the risks as well as the benefits to this, as the supervisor allocated might not have the skills or experience needed and might not be able to meet an SLTs profession-specific concerns. I have observed a lack of clarity about the purpose and nature of professional supervision leading to misassumptions on both sides. Some organisations offer skilled supervision with a psychologist, psychotherapist, another mental health worker or social worker, but they often have no experience of working with SLTs. One SLT I know was told 'well, you just teach skills', which evidenced a lack of understanding of the relational nature of speech and language therapy and left her feeling judged.

I have observed that SLTs may be unfamiliar with the supervisory styles or theoretical approaches they encounter. For example, one supervisee reported hoping for answers and action from a professional supervisor who saw their role as supporting reflection. Conversely, when there is a directive structure for supervision, this does not always match the SLTs need for a reflective space. One SLT I know dreaded supervision because it was process driven and critical, another received emotional support during a crisis, which was then abruptly ended causing resentment.

I notice that group supervision is often offered to staff working with young people with mental health challenges and it can take many forms ranging from non-directive and reflective to the structured discussion of cases. I have been part of group supervision which has been fascinating and insightful, but also where people have felt shamed or persecuted, or where there has been a focus on a few vociferous individuals. In one setting I am aware of, group supervision was avoided because participants found it stressful to sit in silence for long periods.

Misunderstandings and professional supervision of variable quality can be difficult issues to address and questions might be perceived as critical. Supervisors have sometimes not developed effective group management skills or are unable to facilitate discussion about the process of supervision or reflect on their work with openness and curiosity. This latter is a challenge for all of us, can we be 'permeable' practitioners? (The Permeable Practitioner, 2023).

Experience also tells me that there can be blurred boundaries between managerial and professional supervision. For example, a manager offering unexpected and unwelcome 'therapeutic insights' into an SLTs behaviour. I recommend SLTs refer to the RCSLT's 2017 guidance on supervision to support negotiations about whether what is on offer meets their supervision needs.

Many of these issues can be mitigated if the supervisor is experienced and skilful, willing to be open about what they offer and to reflect on how well they can support the supervisee. The next section discusses key considerations in finding such a supervisor.

The value of professional supervision for SLTs in mental health settings

The importance of professional supervision from an SLT

I have noticed that SLTs who are in emerging roles, especially when they are the only SLT in the organisation, often seek professional supervision from an SLT with relevant theoretical and practical knowledge and experience. I think this is because therapists are looking for a shared understanding of the professional role and how this might differ from others. Furthermore, why 'reinvent the wheel' when a supervisor might have faced similar issues? A supervisor may be chosen because of their experience, although an experienced clinician is not necessarily an experienced supervisor. As John Dewey (1933: 78) states, 'we do not learn from experience . . . we learn from reflecting on experience'. So, I would recommend asking about a potential supervisor's level of supervision training and engagement in their own professional supervision and supervision of supervision.

My supervisees often bring systemic issues about the organisations they work for to supervision which underlines the value of having an SLT as a professional supervisor who is external and independent. However, professional supervision from an SLT within an organisation can be useful because of their understanding of the work environment. I also believe that SLTs can gain a lot from cross-professional supervision as it can offer valuable alternate perspectives.

Cultural congruence: personal observations and implications

In my opinion, cultural congruence can be supportive. I notice that SLTs may choose a professional supervisor who is similar to them in terms of ethnicity or gender because the familiarity feels safe. However, in my experience, working with someone who sees things from a different viewpoint can be a rich source of learning for both supervisor and supervisee. I am also aware that I rarely experience prejudice and never experience traumatic microaggressions because of minority, health, disability or neurodivergent status. Consequently, I need to stay alert to such concerns for my supervisees. Although there have been times when my perspective was dismissed by the dominant male culture, even when I have encountered verbal abuse from young people, it was not racist or ableist. As a supervisor, I have been horrified to hear about the discrimination and cruelty experienced by some of my supervisees. Bearing witness to such experiences has helped me recognise my privilege and assumptions; I am part of the majority ethnically and culturally and am fortunate to have trained at a time when university education was essentially free as I could not have accessed it otherwise. My increased awareness of these issues has strengthened my resolve to be an ally alongside supervisees who are marginalised and who experience prejudice or discrimination.

I have observed that working with young people with SEMH brings to the fore issues of intersectionality because multiple factors of disadvantage often impact on young people with mental health challenges. In contrast, SLTs are mostly white, cisgender, middle class women, as are many of the other practitioners who work with them. Although it can be uncomfortable, professional supervision offers opportunities for SLTs and supervisors to consider the often-hidden aspects of their identity that impact on their lives and work, to expose prejudice and increase equality, including in the process of supervision.

Choosing a professional supervisor

In terms of choosing a professional supervisor, I recommend exploring a number of potential supervision options in order to get a clearer sense of how a supervisor works, what they can or cannot offer and if working with them feels comfortable. A non-obligatory introductory session helps both supervisor and supervisee decide if they can work well together. I also believe in the importance of discussions about expectations. For example, supervisees might want a supervisor to provide answers, however professional supervision is a facilitated, reflective process that empowers a supervisee to come to their own understandings and reach their own conclusions.

I believe an important first step in establishing psychological safety in professional supervision is the process of contracting and setting up the supervisory relationship. This allows each participant to discuss what is needed and on offer. This open, honest dialogue enables a negotiated and personalised written contract to be agreed, including discussion of confidentiality, boundaries, content and process as well as how this will be reviewed.

87

Recognising what is needed from professional supervision

Supervisees need to be able to trust their professional supervisor before there can be any learning. An important question to ask is, 'does my supervisor seem to care?' If so, a supervisee is more likely to feel 'seen' and safe and, as the supervisory relationship grows, it might become easier to disclose how challenging this work can be. Research has highlighted the critical role that compassion plays in reducing depression, anxiety and distress and improving wellbeing (Kirby et al., 2017). Consequently, I consider compassion an important component of supervision in mental health settings.

Professional supervision can take many forms and my supervisees have found it useful to address:

- Clinical questions: 'Why is his language more sophisticated when we are listening to music?'
- Service development: 'How can I encourage colleagues to simplify their language?'
- Offloading: 'I think I am annoying!'
- Dilemmas: 'Is screening feasible?'
- Resources: 'How can I develop his narrative skills?'
- Personal and professional development: 'How can I learn more about the co-occurrence of ADHD and Developmental Language Disorder?'
- Wellbeing: 'There's too much to do!'
- Supervision of supervision: 'They are stuck!'

In thinking about what has and has not been useful in professional supervision sessions, we also attend to the process of supervision itself, for example, 'what helped you reach that conclusion?' or 'it seems like that sort of question isn't helpful?' In my experience, the process of reviewing the impact of supervision can help the supervisee clarify their supervision needs. What follows is a discussion of themes that commonly arise in professional supervision.

Understanding the wider context

In my supervision practice, supervisees commonly say they have more difficulty working with other practitioners than they do with the young people.

So, supervision is important for considering the demands on families and other professionals and possibly how SLTs are 'making waves'. I have seen supervision help with reframing others' behaviour more positively, understanding their perspectives and in gaining a deeper understanding of problematic situations.

The supervision I offer also provides opportunities to think about how to respond calmly to perceived threats rather than reacting in ways that can be destructive. There is often reflection on:

- How to 'build bridges' rather than challenge directly
- How to contribute solutions rather than problems
- How to balance autonomy and assertiveness with being a 'team player'
- How to seek feedback
- How to influence key people

The work of Michael West (2021) has personal resonance for me and illustrates the importance of practitioners feeling valued, respected, and supported, both for their own wellbeing and for their effectiveness at work. In my experience, professional supervision can facilitate the recognition when SLTs are not being appropriately valued and supported. No one thrives in an organisation where profit is more important than people, where there is bullying or where staff are seen as expendable. Unfortunately, I observe these are not uncommon experiences. Crucially, professional supervision can provide space for SLTs to reflect on how to advocate for what they need or, if the organisations values do not align with theirs, to recognise the need to move on.

Developing self-awareness

I have seen how professional supervision can help supervisees attune to their own thoughts and feelings, and, as Dan Siegel and Tina Payne Bryson (2011) say, 'name it to tame it'. If there is a word for it, then someone else has experienced it and I know that there can be reassurance in this shared experience. I believe professional supervision can help supervisees recognise assumptions, core beliefs and motivations and how to work in alignment with those that are useful, such as foregrounding our own needs, and reappraise those that do not nourish, for example, ignoring signs of stress. Professional supervision can also help in thinking about healthy and maybe less healthy habits, like saying 'yes' when we mean 'no'. In my personal experience, being really 'seen' and listened to and having thoughts and feelings reflected back in supervision can be both powerful and disturbing, especially if it is unfamiliar. So, although developing self-awareness is vital for flourishing, I think this needs to proceed at a pace that the supervisee is comfortable with.

Personally, professional supervision is important for processing uncomfortable feelings and in recognising overwhelm. Although not recognising the signs of overwhelm can have serious consequences for both the SLT and the quality of their work, it is not always obvious to those experiencing it. Overwhelm/burnout manifests in many ways, including a lack of energy for dealing with change, especially when the changes seem to be relentless, as well as feelings of hopelessness. I notice that some SLTs working with young people with mental health challenges feel that they can function without attending to the emotional impact on themselves. However, supervision can offer an opportunity to recognise when they are overworking or intellectualising the hurt they witness, the repetitive cycles of getting ill or exhausted or taking responsibility for other people's feelings. Hearing a supervisor reflect back, 'you knew you were reaching your limit and you kept going' can be a pivotal moment for the supervisee.

In my experience, professional supervision can help identify 'triggers' and the ability to understand them in others. These triggers frequently evoke stressful events from the past and can be:

- Relational e.g. perceived rejection by a young person or a colleague
- Emotional e.g. sadness as an intolerable emotion
- Autobiographical e.g. Christmas without a family
- Sensory e.g. the smell of aftershave worn by an attacker

If SLTs want to thrive in this field, in my view they must accept their own vulnerability and see it as common humanity, a strength and something to be compassionate about. Expressing vulnerability in professional supervision, either on the part of the supervisor or supervisee, can lead to greater self-understanding and clearer thinking.

Trauma-informed supervision

Many organisations are working toward being 'trauma-informed'. They recognise the signs and symptoms of trauma and overwhelm in young people and practitioners, actively resist re-traumatisation and respond appropriately to those who are struggling (Trauma-Informed Wales, 2022).

Given the high incidence of emotional trauma, arguably supervision for all speech and language therapists must be trauma-informed. Trauma-informed supervision is certainly necessary when working with young people who have experienced abuse or neglect and those with complex challenges including difficulties with mental health and SLCN. I have seen that having a trauma focus in supervision can help with understanding the young people and how their experiences affect those who work and live with them, including SLTs. Trauma-informed supervisors have an understanding and awareness of the signs of trauma, which can range from anger, anxiety and depression to a loss of empathy for oneself and others. Trauma can impact on the body, senses and emotion regulation. Research has shown that trauma-informed supervision can help SLTs recognise how well they are managing in both their work and personal lives and what support is needed to ensure availability to practice (Berger & Quiros, 2014). A supervisee might not realise how stressed they are until they experience strong emotions during supervision. Professional supervision can offer space to explore these emotions, enable self-care and help practitioners to acknowledge when additional support, such as counselling, is required. Supervisors can gain skills in trauma-informed supervision through working in trauma-informed organisations, through receiving this sort of supervision themselves and through trauma-informed supervision training.

I think the idea of 'epistemic trust' is important here: do supervisees' life experiences make it easy for them to trust their supervisor? Professional supervision can facilitate reflection on how the practitioners and the young person's needs are, or are not, being met. For example, whether a therapist's need to 'rescue' clashes with the young person's need to be 'invincible'? I have found supervision to be helpful with accepting that building trusting relationships in the context of trauma can be challenging and take considerable time.

Rough seas make better sailors. Experience has shown me that many skills, including creativity and resourcefulness, can be learned and developed through struggle. Work in this field has driven me towards greater self-awareness and necessitated better self-care for example. The term 'post-traumatic stress disorder' is familiar but 'post-traumatic growth', what can be learnt from very difficult experiences, is less so. Post-traumatic growth is more common than post-traumatic stress disorder if people know it is a possibility and have support to develop it (Wu et al., 2019). I believe trauma-informed supervision can help SLTs recognise the impact of this work, the skills they are developing and how to value them.

Concluding thoughts

I think speech and language therapists can find a powerful 'life belt' in professional supervision, as I have, if they:

- Find a supervisor and supervisory style that works for them
- Receive professional supervision from an SLT to help clarify the SLT role and its' unique contribution, especially in new settings
- Access trauma-informed supervision
- Use supervision to reflect on the impact their work has on them, what is being learnt from it and to plan appropriate self-care

Supervision can help SLTs be more confident in their professional role, can provide validation when uncertain and help develop confidence and assertiveness.

References

Association for Video Interaction Guidance (AVIG) UK (2023). Available online at: www.videointeractionguidance.net/ [Last accessed 2 December 2023].

Berger, R., & Quiros, L. (2014). Supervision for trauma-informed practice. *Traumatology*, 20(4), 296–301. https://doi.org/10.1037/h0099835

Bridger, K. M., Binder, J. F., & Kellezi, B. (2020). Secondary traumatic stress in foster carers: Risk factors and implications for intervention. *Journal of Child and Family Studies*, 29(2), 482–492. https://doi.org/10.1007/s10826-019-01668-2

Dewey, J. (1933). *How We Think: A Restatement of the Relation of Reflective Thinking to the Educative Process*. Chicago, IL: Henry Regnery Company.

Greenberg, D. M., Baron-Cohen, S., Rosenberg, N., Fonagy, P., & Rentfrow, P. J. (2018). Elevated empathy in adults following childhood trauma. *PLOS ONE*, 13(10), e0203886. https://doi.org/10.1371/journal.pone.0203886

Kirby, J. N., Tellegen, C. L., & Steindl. S. R. (2017) A meta-analysis of compassion-based interventions: Current state of knowledge and future directions. *Behaviour Therapy*, 48 (6), 778–792.

Royal College of Speech and Language Therapists Supervision Guidance (2017). Available online at: www.rcslt.org/members/delivering-quality-services/supervision/supervision-guidance/ [Last accessed 2 December 2023].

Siegel, D. J., & Payne Bryson, T. (2011) *The Whole-Brain Child: 12 Revolutionary Strategies to Nurture Your Child's Developing Mind, Survive Everyday Parenting Struggles, and Help Your Family Thrive.* Bantam Books.

The Permeable Practitioner (2023). Available online at: https://thepermeablepractitioner.com/ [Last accessed 2 December 2023].

Trauma-Informed Wales (2022). Available online at: https://traumaframeworkcymru.com/ [Last accessed 2 December 2023].

Turner, H. A., Finkelhor, D., & Ormrod, R. (2010). Poly-victimization in a national sample of children and youth. *American Journal of Preventive Medicine*, 38(3), 323–330. https://doi.org/10.1016/j.amepre.2009.11.012

UK Trauma Council (no date). Available online at: https://uktraumacouncil.org/ [Last accessed 2 December 2023].

West, M. A. (2021) *Compassionate Leadership: Sustaining Wisdom, Humanity and Presence in Health and Social Care.* Swirling Leaf Press. Available online at: www.kingsfund.org.uk/publications/what-is-compassionate-leadership#why-does-compassionate-leadership-matter

Wu, X., Kaminga, A. C., Dai, W., Deng, J., Wang, Z., Pan, X., & Liu, A. (2019). The prevalence of moderate-to-high posttraumatic growth: A systematic review and meta-analysis. *Journal of Affective Disorders*, 243, 408–415. https://doi.org/10.1016/j.jad.2018.09.023

8

The Role of Profession-Specific Supervision and Support in the Safe and Effective Care of Clients in Clinical Settings

Jackie McRae and Kimerley Clarke

Professional supervision is a cornerstone of clinical governance and as such is essential for all clinical roles. We will refer to 'professional supervision' as being profession-specific and including both supervision for clinical care and supervision for professional issues such as dealing with interactions with team members. Clinical governance is defined as 'a framework through which healthcare organisations are accountable for continuously improving the quality of their services and safeguarding high standards of care by creating an environment in which excellence in clinical care will flourish' (Scally & Donaldson, 1998).

'Professional supervision is important in promoting a positive culture of patient safety, continuous quality improvement and lifelong learning as its primary purpose'. (Australian Commission on Safety and Quality in Health Care, 2017). This ensures the safe and effective delivery of care to patients/clients in the context of a range of clinical settings. 'Supervision has been associated with higher levels of job satisfaction, improved retention and staff effectiveness. It is also one way for a provider to fulfil their duty of care to staff' (UK Care Quality Commission, 2013).

This chapter will give some real case examples of where the provision of competent and effective professional supervision helped clinicians to provide excellent and competent clinical care. Conversely, it will also articulate

DOI: 10.4324/9781003301141-8

the implications of not providing supervision to the client, clinician, and organisation. The clinical context of these examples has an international perspective with Jackie McRae discussing the implications for acute hospital care in the UK and Kimerley Clarke outlining the different context from the perspective of acute, community care and private practice in the UK and Australia. Kimerley will also discuss the implications for the provision of professional and clinical supervision of speech and language therapy provided from her experience as a clinical leader in a state-wide government role responsible for speech pathology care in rural and remote contexts in Australia.

Professional standards for supervision have been established as core requirements by a number of international professional speech and language therapy/speech pathology governance organisations as outlined below:

- The UK's Health and Care Professions Council – Speech and Language Therapy Standards of proficiency (2023) states that 'At the point of registration, speech and language therapists must be able to: understand the need for active participation in training, supervision and mentoring in supporting high standards of practice, and personal and professional conduct, and the importance of demonstrating this in practice'.
- Speech Pathology Australia's position statement on professional support, supervision and mentoring (2022) states: 'The process of professional support, especially supervision, facilitates accountability and clinical governance. Professional support can lead to improved outcomes, productivity and job satisfaction, and decreased risk to service users'.
- The Royal College of Speech and Language Therapists (2017) states that 'Supervision has been linked to good clinical governance, by helping to support quality improvement, managing risks, and increasing accountability. By supporting supervision, organisations enable staff to deliver care and treatment safely and to an appropriate standard. A structured and effective system of supervision offers an organisation a rigorous way to support, develop and monitor best practice in their staff group. The appropriate level of resources and time need to be in place to affect this'.
- The American Speech-Language-Hearing Association's speech and language therapy scope of practice (2016) states 'that supervision is integral

in the delivery of communication and swallowing services and advances the discipline. Supervision involves education, mentorship, encouragement, counselling, and support across all supervisory roles'.

In this chapter, we will explore the role of profession-specific supervision when provided in the context of challenging situations for clinicians involved in exploring themes of uncertainty in health care circumstances, the risk of occupational stress and burnout. We will also demonstrate the impact of poor quality, limited or absent supervision on patient outcomes and the positive impact of flexible professional supervision models to support safe and effective clinical practice when a clinician is faced with providing services to a client beyond their scope of experience.

Uncertainty through external circumstances

Uncertainty is common in health care settings and may be present as a result of limitations in skills, issues with competency, challenges with colleagues and complexity of the situation or a new clinical environment. An example is the rapid redeployment of clinical staff into the critical care setting to support the work managing covid-19 patients, as demonstrated in Case study 1. In 2020, the pandemic brought unpredictability to an already challenging healthcare environment. The impact was experienced by all clinical services whether they were directly or indirectly involved in the care of covid-19 cases. Several acute hospital services were designated as 'covid-19 only' services, which shifted staff and resources from other clinical areas into covid-19 care at pace and often without time for broad consultation. In UK based speech and language therapy services, community paediatric and adult teams were instructed to halt or dramatically modify their service provision to minimise risk of virus exposure for both staff and vulnerable patient groups. These staff were then redeployed to support acute services outside of their own clinical specialty. During this time, all usual staff support, and supervisory networks were disrupted. Speech and language therapists (SLTs) who found themselves outside of their normal working environments were rapidly provided with skills training to upskill their basic knowledge and competency with supervision that was focused on service provision rather than professional development, for example a community-based adult clinician being seconded into the acute services to provide services into critical care environments. There was no time to establish new relationships of trust, which restricted honesty and openness that is required when dealing with uncertainty in a new environment. Clinical capability would only be tested in the clinical context and so supervisory oversight was vital to support reflective practice, learning and modification of skills during specific activities.

Case study 1: Critical care in covid times – uncertainty for all

The speech and language therapy team in a metropolitan UK teaching hospital had limited skills and experience in the critical care setting prior to the covid-19 pandemic. In early 2020, the hospital was designated as a regional covid-19 inpatient facility which rapidly admitted hundreds of patients requiring critical care. The team quickly found themselves having to manage large numbers of patients referred with acute covid-19 issues alongside communication and swallowing difficulties. One young gentleman who was referred for assessment had recently been diagnosed with a haematological cancer before contracting covid. He developed respiratory failure and required critical care for ventilation via tracheostomy.

There was huge anxiety and concern amongst SLTs about the risk of spreading the covid virus through aerosol generating procedures, which included airway and swallowing rehabilitation. The team had limited access to training and supervision from a senior speech and language therapist with critical care expertise. The experienced SLT was able to facilitate understanding through supervision of the options available for undertaking a bedside assessment of swallowing This was vital as a baseline to identify impairments to plan an intervention, whilst limiting risk of exposure to the clinician. This evaluation identified that the patients had several cranial nerve impairments, and this helped to set up a targeted rehabilitation programme to improve function of these areas. The SLT undertook joint treatment sessions with the clinical supervisor so that she could be given comprehensive and supportive feedback on her own clinical actions, which increased her insight and confidence. The supervisor was able to ensure that any tracheostomy weaning activity was undertaken in line with infection control demands and emerging evidence, to ensure staff and patient safety was maintained. As speech and language therapy services had not previously been highly involved in the critical care environment, there were differences of opinion with the nursing and medical teams on airway management, weaning processes and frequency of input. Through supervision, the SLT was able to explore feelings of uncertainty safely and as competence grew so did the confidence to explain clinical decisions to the wider team. The patient achieved a positive outcome and was able to resume a full oral diet.

In this case, supervision helped the speech and language therapy team to realise that in times of uncertainty healthcare professionals do not always have definitive answers to manage complex patients, but we can use our existing knowledge and skills as a foundation to explore and evaluate options for interventions. By providing professional supervision any risks can be anticipated and managed thereby maintaining clinical governance.

SLTs working in critical care have been developing their practice in this environment for a number of years, so had some level of familiarity with their roles. These were usually focused on early assessment and rehabilitation as part of a multi-disciplinary team that includes doctors, nurses and other allied health professionals. Supervision has been well established in this clinical setting to ensure safe practices through discussion and reflection. During the Covid-19 pandemic, most swallowing and speech activities had to be modified as they were considered to be aerosol generating procedures that would increase spread of the Covid-19. There was a lack of knowledge of the course of disease and recovery for Covid-19 patients and whether usual clinical interventions would harm or improve patient outcomes. To provide professional support, the Royal College of Speech and Language Therapists (RCSLT) convened an expert advisory panel that met on a regular basis to review current guidance in line with national government advice and generate interim guidance to the membership. As the pandemic was also having international impact, clinical expert SLTs gathered from across the world to agree through consensus, what the role of SLTs in critical care should include (Freeman-Sanderson et al., 2021).

Occupational stress and burnout

SLTs often venture into new settings using their previous knowledge and expertise, however there are likely to always be new or different challenges that need to be explored to deliver interventions safely. These contexts can test SLT's clinical and ethical boundaries, including conflict in relationships with colleagues – particularly those in more established roles. This can lead SLTs to high levels of occupational stress and potential burnout, an example could be advocating for clients/patients with medical colleagues, such as in situations where there is misdiagnosis or absent diagnosis. Some contexts, for example severely understaffed services can also force SLTs to work out-side their scope of practice, which can place their patients or clients at risk of harm. These situations can potentially result in adverse consequences for the SLT such as medico-legal litigation or disbarring from their registered status. Other factors that can influence how SLT's experience occupational stress and potentially burnout can be large, unwieldy, and disorganised work-loads. A recent systematic review found consistent evidence that excessive workloads were correlated with a lack of job satisfaction and an increase in stress and burnout. A lack of professional support also appeared to be cor-related with both stress, burnout and job dissatisfaction (Ewen *et al.*, 2021). The link between improved patient outcomes and supervision is highlighted through the process of early discussion of challenging situations and talking through solutions to resolve dilemmas. A regular, prioritised schedule of supervision establishes open and honest conversations and trusting working relationships, which could prevent occupational stress alongside burnout.

Case study 2: Supervision of a recently qualified SLT in an uncertain situation

Mary had qualified less than a year ago and was working as a sole SLT in a newly multidisciplinary private practice owned by a physiotherapist, Nadia. In Australia, private practices are increasingly being established to take advantage of government funding, designed to boost services to disabled and developmentally delayed clients in the community through client held budgets. Mary was predominantly working with paediatric clients who had developmental delays and communication difficulties, although she did provide services one day per fortnight to adults in a nursing home. Mary had minimal undergraduate experience with complex cases and only one clinical placement in a community adult service where she saw a patient with dysphagia.

Mary's employer, Nadia recognised that Mary required professional supervision to complete her requirements for the Competency Based Occupational Standards for new graduates (Speech Pathology Australia 2017). Therefore, Nadia sought the remote professional supervision services of Kelly, an experienced SLT, to provide supervision for Mary on a twice monthly basis. Mary and Kelly developed a professional supervision agreement to agree the frequency, content, and reporting arrangements of the supervision sessions. Kelly also detailed a safe scope of practice document for Mary's employer, Nadia to cover the first 12–18 months of her role in terms of the complexity and number of clients and context. This document reflected national practice guidelines and covered major speech and language therapy clinical domains such as voice disorders, dysphagia and augmentative and alternative communication (AAC).

Approximately 6 months into the supervision relationship, Mary requested an urgent supervision session where it became apparent that she was distressed about a client that she had recently seen for an initial assessment. Mary reported feeling pressured to see the client as she was told they were a 'complex client with a big funding package' and other clinicians from the practice were also seeing the client.

At the initial assessment, Mary noted that this young child of under 3 years with a significant developmental delay, presented with nasogastric feeding and showed signs of dysphagia. The family were refugees who spoke no English and were living in temporary housing. Mary described that the child's mother had issues with mood and attachment, making no eye contact with Mary or the child. There was no interpreter present, so Mary was only able to glean some information from another child of 11 years old with limited English. Mary told Kelly that she felt very out of her depth with the case and when she discussed her concerns with her line manager and colleagues, they were dismissive of her concerns because of the client's 'big funding package'. Mary became upset and broke down in tears during the supervision session because of how overwhelmed she felt with the responsibilities of dealing with this client. She said to Kelly that 'she was sure that despite of her input the client would die'. Kelly calmly listened and reassured Mary that she had reacted professionally and appropriately and using a mixture of restorative and formative supervision styles (Proctor, 2001), she helped Mary frame her next steps. Firstly, as the client had a nasogastric feeding tube (NGT) in-situ it was likely she was under the local children's specialist hospital. Mary was able to identify the task of connecting with the multi-disciplinary team to establish the degree of clinical risk for the client, especially with the NGT being managed at home whilst the family was in a vulnerable situation. Mary subsequently discovered and brought back to supervision, that the child had two recent hospital admissions for aspiration pneumonia – the last of which had resulted in a 3 week stay in intensive care and endotracheal intubation. The multi-disciplinary team had lost contact with the family on discharge due to their house move and were very concerned about the child's health status and welfare. The children's hospital keyworker also reported that there were significant concerns about the mother's ability to care for the child safely. During a further supervision session, Kelly used a restorative supervision style and assisted Mary to gain more distance and identify that the complexity of this client was outside the scope of Mary's current practice and that her duty of care to the client should be to pass the client's care back to the multidisciplinary team at the Children's hospital. Mary was enabled to define her own stage of development using the previously constructed scope of practice document and plan her feedback about this to her employer, Nadia. She reported that she felt reassured by Kelly's professional supervision which helped her to understand that her distress was linked to her lack of experience and that this would improve over time.

Professional supervision, where the skilled clinical supervisor is matched to the SLT's skill and developmental needs, can assist the SLT to develop skills, confidence, and expertise. This enables them to deal with the full gamut of clinical challenges that can improve their awareness and insight into safe, timely and efficient service delivery. Case study 2 exemplifies how a recently qualified SLT was able to share and process her disturbing experience of a complex case within the context of 'restorative' professional supervision. Through this process she was able to establish clear boundaries around her practice to benefit the safe and effective care and longer-term management of the client and enabled her to build stronger and effective clinical networks with multi-disciplinary colleagues and specialist teams that would potentially help other future clients.

Limited or absent supervision

Examples of limited or poor supervision can be difficult to identify against the many other factors involved in clinical care and staff development. However, situations where SLTs are sent referrals late, as clients are discharged home and they are too busy to do detailed assessments are all too common, as shown in Case study 3. With large and unwieldy caseloads SLTs may only screen for gross impairments or be directed towards a diagnosis by the medical team. Intimidated by external factors such as clinical hierarchies and time pressures to meet deadlines, it may be easier not to ask questions or challenge assumptions. SLTs in busy clinical teams may not be adequately supported through the reflective clinical practice as a team due to workforce pressures or there may be a lack of availability of suitable professional supervision to question their findings in the context of the diagnosis they are given and to explore other possible options.

Case study 3: The implications for safe client care when appropriate professional supervision is not sought or provided

David, an adult client, self-referred to Kathy, a private UK based SLT offering online therapy, due to increased concern about his situation. At the initial contact, he reported that he had recently been discharged from his local hospital following a six-day admission after complaining of speech and swallowing issues. These had been diagnosed by the ear nose and throat (ENT) team as being caused by a severe oral candidiasis infection. The inpatient SLT had also discharged him from her caseload as there was 'no physiological reason for his speech and swallowing issues and that it was mostly caused by anxiety'.

David had provided Kathy with a copy of the original SLT's discharge report, and Kathy was surprised to read that no cranial nerve examination or communication assessment was documented as having taken place during David's six-day admission or post-discharge phone follow-up. However, the discharging SLT had reported that his 'articulation and resonance were altered' and 'this appeared to be related to reduced tongue movement'. Despite this, she had not questioned the diagnosis of oral candidiasis as an improbable cause. Kathy suspected that this lack of questioning of the medical diagnosis could be due to clinical inexperience, intimidation within the team dynamic, pressure to discharge the patient to free up a bed, unwieldy caseloads and the lack of professional supervision. David had been discharged from speech and language therapy following a phone review, with a recommendation to seek psychological help for his anxiety despite reporting his ongoing inability to eat soft consistency diet and routinely coughing on thin fluids.

David reported that he now felt extremely anxious as his speech and swallowing issues were ongoing and he was seeking access to a private psychologist to help with his anxiety but stated that waiting lists were long. He was able to take sufficient fluids but was not able to eat any food and had lost a significant amount of weight in the last three weeks since his discharge from hospital.

Kathy undertook a preliminary oral-motor assessment and discovered significant neurological bulbar signs including severe hypernasality, diminished cough reflex and bilateral ptosis (inability of close his eyes properly). David's speech was only 50% intelligible in conversation due to moderately severe dysarthria, but no cognitive impairment was apparent. Kathy established that there had been a gradual onset of these neurological symptoms over the last two to three months, which presented with speech and swallowing difficulties. This meant it predated the candidiasis infection, that had been mistakenly identified as the cause. Kathy advised David to present to an emergency department of a different hospital as soon as possible after suspecting he may have an undiagnosed progressive neurological disease with bulbar features. Kathy was able to reassure David that his neurological symptoms were real, making his anxiety a perfectly reasonable reaction. Subsequently, David contacted Kathy to inform her that he had been admitted to hospital and formally diagnosed with Myasthenia Gravis and provided with treatment. Kathy did not see David for any further input as his care was being provided by a specialist multidisciplinary team.

If appropriate and skilled professional supervision had been provided to the initial SLT identified in Case study 3, reflective clinical practice could have enabled a different decision-making process and the client would have had a very different experience of his first health-care episode. Certainly, at the time of the self-referral, the client was at significant risk of malnutrition, aspiration, and potential respiratory complications in addition to significant psychological harm, which would have been compounded over time. Fortunately for this client, he had sufficient courage to seek help from a private SLT despite the poor experience he had had during his first admission and the length of wait for public outpatient health service assessment. Following the correct signposting by the private therapist, ultimately his health outcomes were much more positive with his ongoing care being provided by an experienced SLT, who is a part of a multidisciplinary neurological specialist service.

Professional supervision to support safe and effective clinical practice

The provision of professional supervision in the aforementioned scenarios is essential and should be tailored to the needs of the clinician and the context of their professional role. Professional supervision here is differentiated from the functions of line management, which is often related to employment and workplace matters without clinical content. Professional supervision should be a safe space for discussion, encouraging the development, maturation and maintenance of clinical reasoning and skills. The goal would be to support the application of skills and knowledge from assessment and the understanding of universal interventions to then create bespoke interventions to suit client needs, wishes and the client's social and clinical context. For this to be maximally effective, it is important for all clinicians including sole practitioners, to have self-awareness of their own competency level and openly with honesty, seek and engage in the supervisory process.

Professional supervision should be an established part of every clinician's career, regardless of their level of expertise, and recognises that dilemmas and challenges are integral to career progression.

There are options for the type of supervision and how it is accessed as a more senior clinician. It may be focused on professional development rather than clinical development or more specifically on specialist skills development, such as using new diagnostic equipment or digital-based interventions. Supervision for more experienced clinicians may be with a colleague or colleagues in the context of formal, structured peer supervision where the clinicians benefit from the facilitated opportunity to share scenarios for further discussion, catharsis, re-framing, and problem solving. An alternative process that provides valuable insights for senior staff has been reverse mentoring, whereby junior or less experienced staff can discuss their perceptions of processes or situations from their perspectives, that highlight hierarchical barriers and enable new solutions to be considered. There are also scenarios where professional supervision can be provided by colleagues external to one's own profession as they may be familiar with the organisation or client group and increase one's own awareness of the wider context. This is especially of benefit to increase recognition of issues of inclusion and diversity and find solutions that are immediately translatable into practice.

Case study 4: Remote professional supervision model of supporting a less experienced colleague with a highly complex client

Daniela was a SLT with approximately 1.5 years' experience, who worked in a large Australian rural health organisation that had a robust professional supervision policy with access to regular planned professional supervision with her on-site senior SLT. Daniela had a 2.5-year-old child on her caseload in a remote, rural location, with a highly complex medical history and supportive family. The child had a tracheostomy tube in situ due to a severe respiratory illness following an admission to intensive care in the preceding 12 months. He was being cared for at home by his family and receiving a complex package of care through live-in nurses 24 hours per day. A modified barium swallow at a specialist metropolitan hospital during his initial inpatient admission, confirmed aspiration on all consistencies, he received all his nutrition through a gastrostomy tube. His tracheostomy tube cuff remained fully inflated to protect his airway from aspiration, leaving him with no ability to use his voice for communication. He showed a mild general developmental delay consistent with his medical history. Daniela's focus had been to support communication attempts using augmentative and alternative means of communication such as Makaton and picture exchange systems, however the child was extremely hard to engage with these systems. His mother reported extreme behavioural disturbance at home both with his parents and other siblings, and that he often attempted oral communication but became extremely frustrated and angry when he could not be understood by his communication partners.

Daniela's regular clinical supervisor agreed that her client was very complex and in fact she herself did not have the clinical expertise to provide supervision to support Daniela's work with him. The professional lead for the speech and language therapy service was asked to provide supplementary 1:1 professional supervision with Daniela to manage this case. This colleague was located a distance away, so supervision was set up to include one face-to-face joint clinical assessment and ongoing remote support via videoconferencing. This allowed regular contact to develop a safe treatment plan in partnership with the specialist hospital tracheostomy nurse specialist, local nursing and medical team to support the child and family. A clear management plan was established to document any adverse responses to a partial cuff deflation programme and identify the child's tolerance. Daniela reported in her usual supervision sessions that she was feeling more confident having the support of a more experienced colleague in managing a patient with such a complex clinical presentation. She reported that she had identified a gap in her knowledge and that she was doing reading to further develop her knowledge of tracheostomy management.

A positive outcome resulted in the child being able to achieve leak speech straight away with no evidence of laryngeal pathology. His communication, behaviour and relationships with the family subsequently improved significantly as his frustration subsided. Other benefits were observed with saliva swallowing and a repeat modified barium swallow was planned for his next hospital visit to ascertain if any improvements in swallowing function for food and fluids had also occurred.

Case study 4 demonstrates an organisation that is serious about professional supervision and clinical growth and skill development, leading to positive impact for the client and potentially offers enormous cost savings to the wider health care economy. The enhancement of skills, confidence and job satisfaction developed by the supervisee SLT through her supported care with this client was also invaluable. An organisation where the hierarchy allows for a clinical specialist to provide tailored content-rich professional supervision to a SLT, alongside their regular professional supervision, is one where genuine learning and support for high quality client care is the major goal.

Value of organisational support for supervision in the context of good clinical governance

A healthcare organisation committed to clinical governance is one that prioritises and ensures that professional supervision is of high quality, occurs regularly and is supported by organisational policies and procedures that includes professional supervision for staff at all levels of seniority. Policies should clearly articulate a minimum standard or framework of professional supervision both in quality and frequency and establish documentation that records metrics of supervisory practice. (Snowdon et al., 2020; Turnbull et al., 2009). Critical to this functioning well is a policy that clearly articulates the roles of supervisee, supervisor, line manager and a lead for professional supervision who oversees the professional standards in the supervisory process. This includes training through standardised modules to establish clear and unambiguous expectations of what professional supervision is for all professional employees. Training should be available to any new or existing employees who receive or provide professional supervision and support the clinical governance process. Professional leads should be responsible for oversight of professional supervision for all team members, particularly for sole practitioners or where the clinicians receive line management from staff outside of their profession. Additionally, consideration should be given to tailored shorter term supervision designed to help develop a clinician's skills or expertise in a particular clinical specialism.

Ideally, the supervisee should have sufficient self-awareness about their requirements for building a trusting and meaningful supervisory relationship and this subsequently would influence the choice of supervisor to best meet their needs. In turn, the supervisor should be capable of utilising multiple styles of supervision to facilitate and support the supervisee to maximise their professional learning and growth. Supervisors should have the opportunity to grow their supervisory skill base through training and their own self-reflection facilitated by supervision too. The healthcare organisation should encourage robust and transparent evaluation of the application of their supervision policy and procedures through tools such as 360-degree evaluation or the use of published supervision evaluation scales such as the Manchester Clinical Supervision Scale (Winstanley, 2000). All these measures are essential to maintaining a tangible and robust supervision framework that is genuinely embedded as a core standard of the organisation's quality clinical governance policy.

Concluding thoughts

In this chapter, we have explored the essential role of professional supervision to develop and maintain safe clinical practices. This process should be supported by professional leads and organisational policies to ensure a framework for good practice is embedded in daily activity. The case studies demonstrate a variety of scenarios where professional supervision was beneficial to care and preventing risks. We caution against quick and uninformed decisions as these carry consequences for our clients and our practice. These principles are important throughout our career pathway and staff at all levels of seniority should ensure that supervision is mandated in their practice.

References

American Speech-Language-Hearing Association. (2016) Speech and Language Therapy scope of practice. Retrieved from www.asha.org/policy/sp2016-00343/

Australian Commission on Safety and Quality in Health Care. (2017). National Safety and Quality Health Service Standards. Sydney: ACSQHC. Retrieved from www.safetyandquality.gov.au/sites/default/files/migrated/National-Safety-and-Quality-Health-Service-Standards-second-edition.pdf

Care Quality Commission. (2013) Supporting information and guidance: Supporting effective clinical supervision. Retrieved from https://work-learn-live-blmk.co.uk/wp-content/uploads/2018/04/CQC-Supporting-information-and-guidance.pdf

Ewen, C., Jenkins, H., Jackson, C., Jutley-Neilson, J., & Galvin, J. (2021). Well-being, job satisfaction, stress and burnout in speech-language pathologists: A review. *Int J Speech Lang Pathol*, 23(2), 180–190. https://doi.org/10.1080/17549507.2020.1758210

Freeman-Sanderson, A., Ward, E. C., Miles, A., de Pedro Netto, I., Duncan, S., Inamoto, Y., McRae, J., Pillay, N., Skoretz, S. A., Walshe, M., Brodsky, M. B., & Group, C.-S. G. (2021). A Consensus Statement for the Management and Rehabilitation of Communication and Swallowing Function in the ICU: A Global Response to COVID-19. *Arch Phys Med Rehabil*, 102(5), 835–842. https://doi.org/10.1016/j.apmr.2020.10.113

Health and Care Professions Council. (2023). Standards of proficiency – Speech and Language Therapists. HCPC. Retrieved 1 October 2024 from www.hcpc-uk.org/resources/standards/standards-of-proficiency-speech-and-language-therapists/

Proctor, B. (2001). 'Training for the supervision alliance: Attitude, skills and intention' in J. Cutcliffe, T.Butterworth and B. Proctor, (eds) *Fundamental Themes in Clinical Supervision*. London: Routledge

Royal College of Speech and Language Therapists. (2017). Supervision: Information for Speech and Language Therapists. RCSLT. Retrieved 1 February 2024 from www.rcslt.org/members/delivering-quality-services/supervision

Scally, G., & Donaldson, L. J. (1998). Clinical governance and the drive for quality improvement in the new NHS in England. *BMJ*, 317(7150), 61–65. https://doi.org/10.1136/bmj.317.7150.61

Snowdon, D. A., Sargent, M., Williams, C. M., Maloney, S., Caspers, K., & Taylor, N. F. (2020). Effective clinical supervision of allied health professionals: a mixed methods study. *BMC Health Services Research*, 20(1). https://doi.org/10.1186/s12913-019-4873-8

Speech Pathology Australia. (2017). Competency Based Occupational Standards for Speech Pathologists: Entry Level. The Speech Pathology Association of Australia Limited. Retrieved 1st January, 2022 from www.speechpathologyaustralia.org.au/public/libraryviewer?ResourceID=77

Speech Pathology Australia. (2022). Position Statement: Professional support, supervision and mentoring. Retrieved 1 February 2024 from work-learn-live-blmk.co.uk/wp-content/uploads/2018/04/CQC-Supporting-information-and-guidance.pdf

Turnbull, C., Grimmer-Somers, K., Kumar, S., May, E., Law, D., & Ashworth, E. (2009). Allied, scientific and complementary health professionals: A new model for Australian allied health. *Australian Health Review*, 33(1), 27. https://doi.org/10.1071/ah090027

Winstanley, J. (2000). Manchester Clinical Supervision Scale. *Nurs Stand*, 14(19), 31–32.

Supervision
A Personal and Professional Perspective

9

Lorraine Maher-Edwards

In this chapter, I draw upon many experiences of supervision from a number of perspectives. Firstly, I have been client for both stammering therapy and psychological therapy throughout my life. Secondly, as a legal requirement practising as a counselling psychologist in both the National Health Service (NHS) and private practice, I have received supervision throughout my career and have supervised many qualified and trainee psychologists. In addition, as a member of the stammering community, I have received supervision when mentoring adults and young people who stammer.

In this chapter I foreground my position as client, but as someone who also has experience of being both clinician and supervisor, to provide a unique lens on how important supervision is to safe and effective practice and the benefits of this for the client. In preparation for this piece one of the challenges was the invisibility of supervision to the client. As client, I have never known what supervision my therapists have had and what influence that may have had on the work; however, I have been able to draw upon my clinical experience to wonder. Below are some reflections on therapy experiences from my place as client who is also a clinician and supervisor.

I remember in my younger adult years, as a person with an interiorised stammer accompanied by high levels of anxiety, I was intent on finding a way to control both. By which I mean I was keen to find a technique or skill to get rid of what I perceived as weaknesses of will; in the meantime, whilst waiting for the answer to the problem to reveal itself, I felt the only option was to hide both my dysfluency and my anxiety. In retrospect, given where I was in my journey towards acceptance of stammering, this does not surprise me. The societal context was one where fluency was prized alongside being confident, extrovert and keeping your emotions in check. No one

DOI: 10.4324/9781003301141-9

could say I did not try. I was a master at avoidance of speaking situations and word switching and was working my way through potential techniques, like breathing, mindfulness meditation, and telling myself to just stop being anxious and relax. My General Practitioner (GP) had recommended psychological therapy to help with my anxiety and in particular Cognitive Behaviour Therapy (CBT); I felt sure if my anxiety was 'sorted out' my stammering would fall away too.

My therapist was kind and caring and wanted to help. However, the psychological perspective from which she came (CBT), for me, played into my agenda of control. Absorbing societal messages about positivity as a matter of will and stammering as a problem to be fixed, I was sure that I was the problem. Stopping my negative thinking, being more positive and facing situations I was avoiding became the perceived way to the holy grail. I have no doubt my psychotherapist had my best interests at heart, but in retrospect I can see that the therapy just became another ineffective tool to try and help me control my speech and anxiety, reinforcing self-stigma and ultimately bringing a sense of renewed failure that yet again I had not been able to crack it.

Supervision plays a crucial role in helping clinicians to be able to observe and notice the therapeutic process. Key to this is using their own experience as useful information in understanding the client's process and how that may be playing out in their daily lives. Did my therapist have a space to do this? Did she have somewhere she was able to step out of the CBT model and notice that the process that was playing out in therapy *was* the thing that I needed to be able to observe and work on? To be supported to compassionately confront how the pursuit of control was at the cost of self-acceptance and ultimately was bringing more suffering. To see that this was not a problem located within me but rather an interaction between me and my learning history within a particular culture and society. One that was characterised by narratives around fluency as necessary for effective communication and difficult emotions like anxiety as problems to be sorted. I wonder if I was the only one in the room feeling a sense a failure, like I just had to try harder? The role of clinicians as helpers within a system built upon a medical model emphasises problem-solving, behaviour change and treatment of 'problems'. Clinical interactions whereby clients do not make what we see as necessary changes can feel very deskilling for therapists; if the clinician is not supported to step back and observe both their own and their clients' narratives at play, they can find themselves right in the soup along with the client. This particular experience for me as a client felt confusing and I left with an unspoken feeling I had failed at the therapy.

I hold this experience alongside a later experience when, as a counselling psychologist in training, I had a requirement to have my own personal therapy. I remember my shock when, after a few sessions, this therapist, both kind and firm, pointed out that from where she was sitting, I was going around in well-worn circles, keeping safe behind carefully crafted defences all the while avoiding what really needed to be looked at and felt. Of course, this in-session process was precisely what was going on outside therapy. I can only imagine that it must have taken courage to be so bold to tackle so directly what was an unhelpful process playing out and I did not thank her for it right there and then! With time though I learned that this was an expression of compassion, allowing me to be where I was *and*, from there, doing what was needed to help me to find a way to become unstuck, she was willing to step out of the content and point to the process even when it felt uncomfortable, all in the service of helping me. This ability to slow down and with mindful awareness notice the process, so called compassionate metacommunication, is developed and honed in the safe space that is supervision.

The aforementioned straight-talking therapist continued to challenge me to step into painful territory that I had previously been avoiding, most notably the devastating sudden loss of my Dad. I met her almost a year after his death, a year during which I had hardly spoken about him or his death, so painful it was to even name. As children we develop ways of understanding the world that make sense to us and allow for the safety of a sense of rationality, fairness and predictability. Whilst we might feel we 'know' things can change in a moment; on a deep level we cling to an assumption that it will not. With my Dad's death my world assumptions were shattered, an experience that was highly threatening and destabilising, bringing emotions that felt too big to have or express. The lack of narratives around death in society often reinforces keeping emotions in check and getting on with things. I felt intuitively that this therapist was able to contain my emotions and knowing she was supported to do this in her supervision allowed me to be unburdened by fears about the impact of my emotions on the other. This therapist was a fiercely compassionate witness, she did not look away from my grief but instead stayed present, curious and non-judgemental. This allowed me to learn that these were experiences I could have alongside my other life experiences.

Working in healthcare can be tough and clinicians need to have within their own repertoire the ability to notice and skilfully respond to their own emotions and those that resonate with the clients'. Supervision might involve understanding how clinical work is bringing up unresolved experiences for the therapist. Exploring and working with emotion in supervision also provides the therapist with an experience of how this can skilfully be carried out. More broadly, supervision can help clinical staff to acknowledge and understand the impact of their work on them, personally and professionally and provides an important space where self-care is always on the agenda, reducing risk of burnout and compassion fatigue. Studies have shown (Bond & Bunce, 2003; Iglesias et al., 2010) that clinicians who tend to avoid or suppress difficult feelings are more at risk of burnout, which is characterised by detachment and avoidant coping. Conversely, effective clinicians can remain in contact with their own emotional experience, and this will facilitate their work; however, this emotional availability also represents a vulnerability and clinical staff need a safe space to tread that line.

Clinicians in healthcare are often drawn to these professions out of commitment to care for others, to hold their hands during their most difficult moments, to support them to make important changes in their lives, often hugely courageous, terrifying changes. The topography might look different in the psychological therapist's room, the physiotherapy consultation or the speech and language therapist's office in school, but the work resonates with clinicians, as they support clients to navigate difficulties and find ways to live full and meaningful lives often in the face of great challenge. Dependent on your profession, this might be supporting them to express their feelings to their loved ones, take their first step following a devastating accident or to re-find their voice post-stroke. When I embarked on my training journey as a psychologist, I anticipated the joy, the reward, the warm glow of knowing I had touched someone's life in a meaningful way, however in my experience what clinicians do not come prepared for is the difficult feelings and thoughts that they will encounter regularly in their work, from frustration, helplessness, compassion fatigue to shame and despair. Whilst these feelings remain a part of the process, supervision plays a huge role in helping clinicians to make sense of these feelings and hold themselves with kindness and self-compassion as they tread this road. Having experienced therapy from both sides, feeling psychologically safe in supervision allows a mirroring containment for the client. Clients know when their therapist is supported in this way by a supervisor, this knowing may not be explicit but will be felt in the room. Safe and effective supervision scaffolds the therapeutic work, enabling both safety and freedom for client and therapist.

References

Bond, F. W. & Bunce, D. (2003) The role of acceptance and job control in mental health, job satisfaction, and work performance. *Journal of Applied Psychology*, 88(6), 1057–1067.

Iglesias, M., de Bengoa Vallejo, R. & Fuentes, P. (2010) The relationship between experiential avoidance and burnout syndrome in critical care nurses: A cross-sectional questionnaire survey. *Journal of Nursing Studies*, 47, 30–37.

From Permafrost to Permeability

10

Supervision as the Foundation of Professional and Public Safety

Deborah Harding

I often describe supervision as fundamental for professional and public safety in healthcare, but this has not always been the case. Here, I describe my supervision 'thawing'. I share ideas about the inevitable uncertainties which healthcare practitioners experience and a cluster of behaviours which can help practitioners to navigate uncertainty. These ideas developed through my PhD (Harding 2019) and have been elaborated in work with the National Health Service (NHS) and as a healthcare educator in the United Kingdom (UK).

Supervision permafrost

I qualified as a speech and language therapist (SLT) in 1990. I focused on working with adults with neurogenic communication problems. I recall little, if any, supervision-focused teaching in my training. In an era when the value of supervision was only just beginning to be discussed in UK healthcare, this is perhaps unsurprising.

In my first job I was often the only SLT onsite. Fortunately, I worked with experienced, multi-professionals who looked out for me. I did not recognise it at the time, but now wonder if I might have felt greater security with more readily accessible profession-specific support to guide me through the 'transition shock' (Duchscher 2009) which can accompany being newly qualified.

My next job brought access to a bigger and more accessible team of SLTs who guided my subsequent professional steps. I am not sure we called it

DOI: 10.4324/9781003301141-10

supervision but the opportunities to talk through clinical situations, observe and be observed, built my confidence as an SLT. A later change of manager connected me with someone who explicitly referred to and was enthusiastic about supervision. I felt less persuaded.

I veered off into management. I became responsible for in-patient, community and out-patient services and for the multi-professional workforce and budget necessary to deliver these. Supervision continued, often with, for and from other professions and accompanied by a mix of good and less good experiences. I had valuable leadership supervision, notably with a director whose background was in occupational therapy. I also augmented my professional development and sense-making through action learning sets (Revans, 2011) and with peers who shared an interest in personal construct psychology (Kelly, 1963). Eventually, work/life imbalance prompted some 'fantasy job hunting'. I joined a university physiotherapy department which was building a team to deliver a multi-professional master's programme. It seemed like a good fit and an opportunity to share my multi-professional leadership experience. Moving from health to academia was like getting into a cognitive spa. It prompted me to reflect on my taken-for-granted health service practices and to explore research, opinion and theory. One taken-for-granted practice which started to bother me was supervision.

Supervision paradox and the search for answers

The Health and Care Professions (HCPC) standards of proficiency for practice state, both then and now, that registrants should:

> understand the need for active participation in training, supervision and mentoring in supporting high standards of practice, and personal and professional conduct, and the importance of demonstrating this in practice.
>
> (HCPC 2023, p. 9)

Why then did I observe and experience supervision getting cancelled when colleagues and I felt pressured in practice? Why did we argue for protected supervision time if we cancelled or neglected to schedule so freely? Why did developing as a supervisor get so little attention? The master's students also recognised these paradoxes. I was feeling increasingly chilly and uncertain about supervision and turned to the academic evidence-base for clarity.

Turning to the literature

I found a surprising lack of consistency in the literature but it did reflect some of my uncertainties and demonstrated I was not the only person looking for clarity. There was a lengthy history of debate, which Lynch, Happell and Sharrock (2008) found extends to definition, aims, models and purpose of supervision. Their review also identified a link with governance and the use by some, of the term 'snoopervision' indicating a sense of surveillance which others have also debated (Gilbert 2001; Clouder and Sellars 2004; Rolfe and Gardener 2006). Gilbert's (2001) view that supervision and reflective practice have become hegemonic practices which are less benign than those who promote them claim initially startled me. However, as I continued exploring, I found myself more empathetic to his suggestion that the presumed benefits and underpinning assumptions about supervision seemed largely unchallenged and seldom subject to the sort of critical debate which is familiar in contemporary evidence-informed healthcare practice. These themes mirrored my own early career unease that supervision was about checking up on me. Talking through, not only my caseload but also how things were for me felt intrusive and uncomfortable. With limited prior exposure to supervision, I reflect that I equated early supervision encounters with the role play scenarios I had found uncomfortable as a novice SLT in counselling skills courses. My less positive constructs of counselling role play perhaps coloured my supervision sense-making.

When I was newly qualified, I was bursting to land my new knowledge and wanted space to do so without any sense of someone checking up on me. What might have been helpful to 'novice me' would have been exposure to and insight from models and theories of supervision. Yet it was not until I was immersed in my PhD some 20 years after qualifying, that I began to consider how models and theories can support effective supervision. I started to ask myself how I could have been having and providing supervision for so long with such limited awareness. In my research, I asked allied health professionals (AHPs) how they acquired supervisor knowledge and skills. Like me, few had read any publications or research about supervision. Most picked up their knowledge and skills vicariously, replicating good experiences and avoiding replicating the less favourable ones. This apparent willingness to leave supervisor development to chance was consistent with my NHS management recollection that requests from staff to attend supervision-related professional development were vanishingly rare. Given the HCPC expectations about engagement in supervision, this troubled me. It seemed unthinkable that as registrants we would be similarly casual about clinical development.

Forming a hypothesis

As I began my PhD, I was forming a hypothesis that tendencies to neglect development of supervisor capability and to postpone or cancel supervision indicated that colleagues were at best ambivalent about this aspect of practice. Yet there was a paradox because colleagues spoke about the need to protect time for supervision. I was interested to hear what it was that made something so readily abandoned, also something to protect. With an acknowledged and sizeable productivity challenge in healthcare (Appleby, Galea and Murray, 2014) employers were and remain preoccupied with client or patient facing activity. Without further insights about supervision's value, it felt tricky to argue the case for protected time, even though supervision was beginning to catch employer's attention with responsibilities for supervision changing following Kirkup's (2015) report on maternity and neonatal services in a UK NHS provider. As the only health profession to have mandated supervision dating back to the 1902 Midwives Act, it was apparent that this legal imperative did not prevent the unthinkable happening. Mandatory supervision for midwives ended and responsibility for workplace supervision transferred from statute to employer. So, I embarked on my PhD not with an intention to prove the worth of supervision but to gain insights from practitioners about its possible value. I remained concerned about issues of power, privilege and surveillance (Harding, 2019, p. 279) and was open to the possibility that I might discover a form of 'Emperor's New Clothes'. However, if value could be demonstrated, that might be persuasive, not only for practitioners but also for employers and policy makers.

Inevitable practice uncertainties: a prompt to learn.

I began my research by asking AHPs to pick photographs which might tell me something about supervision. They spoke about the images they selected, providing stories from supervisor and supervisee standpoints. They described good, poor and seemingly toxic experiences. What I heard most of all were practitioners talking about their uncertainties, who they can share them with and how to navigate them. These AHPs had been qualified for between six months and 30 years. Without exception they described uncertainties, demonstrating that this is a career-long phenomenon. I became interested in practice uncertainties, how practitioners spotted them, who they shared them with and what helped them to make sense of and address them.

I returned to the literature with a different focus. Instead of searching for what had been written about supervision, my search terms were about uncertainty and learning. Of course, recognising uncertainty in healthcare is not new. Fox (1957) called for medical education to include training for uncertainty, drawing attention to inevitable uncertainties arising from the limits to a practitioner's own knowledge, the limits of what is known or a combination of these. There is also nothing new in suggesting that however experienced we are, it is wise to look out for uncertainties, acknowledge them and seek to attend to their implications. Eraut (1994) describes human experts as fallible, with the potential for knowledge and skills to decay, become outdated or less relevant. He suggests that a wise professional makes time for regular reflection and self-evaluation which, combined with an ongoing willingness to learn from colleagues, ensures the professional retains critical control over aspects of practice which have become intuitive and taken for granted. Dall'Alba and Barnacle (2015) draw attention to the relationship between uncertainty and established professional practices and, in earlier work, Dall'Alba (2009) discusses how becoming a professional (not just in healthcare) involves both the acquisition of knowledge and skills as well as developing ways of being. Schön's (1983) influential writing about reflection identifies uncertainty as a prompt to reflect and for Webster-Wright (2010) uncertainty is a precursor for authentic professional learning; learning that is significant and meaningful because the practitioner cares about and cares to resolve that uncertainty.

The AHPs' stories represented much of this existing theory and opinion. They described career-long uncertainty. They recognised their own fallibility and engaged in continuous professional development activities which they identified as offering promising ways to navigate and potentially resolve their uncertainties. When, and only when practitioners felt they had a trusting and collaborative relationship with a supervisor, they shared practice concerns in scheduled supervision as part of wider continuing professional development endeavours. These wider endeavours include but are not limited to engaging with the published literature, being part of professional social media groups, attending courses, joining learning sets, shadowing, being observed or working collaboratively with a more experienced colleague or supervisor. AHPs' accounts expanded my understanding about the potential value of supervision as a component of practitioner learning in, for and from practice. Under favourable conditions, supervision provides an opportunity for practitioners to check, assure and if necessary, adjust so that they feel and are safe in practice. Supervision began to seem like an important aspect of practitioner capability, well-being and a mechanism for the maintenance and protection of a hard-won professional registration. By implication, supervision was also vital for public safety as it is reasonable to assume that a safe practitioner provides safe care. I was beginning to thaw.

Thinking about categories of practice uncertainty in supervision

Initially informed by AHPs' accounts and subsequently through my ongoing work across the health workforce, I observe that practitioner uncertainties are messy, overlapping and often ill-defined. I propose that when we are working out how to navigate uncertainties, in supervision for example, it is helpful to think about them as three intertwined categories: Practice Demands, Platform for Practice and Socio-Professional, as illustrated in Table 10.1.

As a supervisor, an educator and in my policy-influencing roles, I and others find these categories helpful. I acknowledge synergies with formative, normative and restorative dimensions of supervision (e.g., Proctor 2008, p. 7):

- Formative: Supporting learning and development, knowledge and skills
- Normative: Supporting maintenance of standards of practice and care
- Restorative: Supporting professional well-being in practice and the impact of practice demands

Table 10.1 Indicative categories of practitioner uncertainty

Categories of practice uncertainty		
Practice demands	Platform for practice Knowledge + skills + experiences (in and out of practice) + personal factors	Socio-professional
• Feeling less efficient than colleagues • Being new to a role or specialty – feeling daunted • Feeling the burden of one's own expectations • Burden arising from perceived expectations of others • Impact of supervisor being on leave • A new or unanticipated change in practice, such as the impact of a pandemic	• Professional knowledge and skills • Experiences in different specialities e.g. in developmental rotational posts • Previous work experiences in a contrasting job • Knowing a patient in another context • Impact and/or relevance of out of work experiences; a health condition, unwell relative etc. • Knowledge and skills gained outside of practice: a previous career, being a sports coach, a board position with a not-for-profit organisation • Preferences and personal characteristics: working to a plan, happy to experiment, creative, cautious, etc.	• Having a recognised professional role • Being at different stages of professional development/different career points • Perceptions of peers • Being different from others in your team: race, gender, sexuality, age, neurodiversity, etc. • Perceptions of more experienced colleagues • Perceptions of other professional groups • Being visible – to patients, carers, colleagues • Having expectations of self (in practice and beyond) • Being in a non-traditional role

I often work with both ideas together. For example, enthusiastic, newly qualified me was focused on augmenting my novice practitioner platform for practice to meet the practice demands encountered each day; 'how do I tick off my competences and get through my caseload?' Supervision could have provided opportunities to check whether I was doing what was expected and to required standards (normative) or where I needed to gain more knowledge, for example by attending training in specific aspects of practice (formative). Professional transitions, like the progression from student to qualified professional, involve landing knowledge and skills safely in practice but are accompanied by socio-professional adjustments; 'do I look like a therapist, am I fitting in with the team, do patients trust me?' There are restorative benefits associated with formative and normative assurance from the supervisor, for example, about the application of knowledge or ways to manage practice demands such as prioritising or time management. There is additional restorative value when supervision provides safe opportunities to share the anticipated and unanticipated emotional demands encountered daily.

Unpicking the dimensions of an uncertainty: where to begin?

In practice, it is not always easy to spot what will help to identify the core source of an uncertainty or the most promising course of action to resolve it. This is where the platform for practice idea is valuable. The template (Figure 10.1) can help to structure self-assessment or supervisee/supervisor discussion. It can be used to think about a role, a point in the career path, requirements for a future career path, a specific practice encounter and so on. As a supervisor, I might ask a supervisee to think about an issue in terms of these headings ahead of supervision and/or work through it together.

Figure 10.2 is a retrospective analysis for a time when I worked in neurosurgery. I had some years' experience but was more comfortable working with patients on the ward than in intensive care.

This analysis demonstrates multiple contributory factors for my uncertainty. I suggest there is a need for both opportunistic and scheduled in-practice supervision (Rolfe 2011) as well as scheduled time for supervision away from the practice setting to support more private reflective learning. Formative and normative knowledge and skills' gaps might be addressed through familiarisation with the intensive care environment, some joint working or direct in-practice supervision with a more experienced colleague. Away from the clinical environment, supervision might guide me to work through my perfectionist traits and risk aversion, and potentially explore whether more specific psychological support could be helpful in working through the distress linked to a personal experience of intensive care.

Knowledge	Skills	Experience	Behaviours, characteristics, personal qualities and preferences
Use this space to capture all the different kinds of knowledge here: • Clinical • Technical • Operational Think about the things you put on your Curriculum Vitae (CV) but think specifically about the knowledge you have acquired	Use this space to capture all the different kinds of skills here: • Clinical • Interpersonal • Technical • Operational Again, your CV might help but really focus on the skills	Use this space to capture your professional and work experiences	Be honest with yourself about helpful and less helpful behaviours … organised, a bit last minute, friendly ….
		Use this space to capture personal experiences which might influence your practice. Include things that augment your practice as well as things that might be challenges. Anything from being a sportscoach to being a patient.	… and characteristics and personal qualities … private, chatty, perfectionist, approachable, short-tempered … … and preferences … early bird, being active, avoiding conflict, working shifts, working regular hours …

Figure 10.1 Template to support platform for practice discussions

(Harding 2023a)

Knowledge	Skills	Experience	Behaviours, characteristics, personal qualities and preferences
• Confident about neuro' knowledge • Confident about assessment and management knowledge for speech and language in ward setting • Confident about knowledge of swallowing problems post neurosurgery • Limited knowledge of swallow assessment for patients with tracheostomy • Knowledge of staff on neurosurgery ward but don't know the intensive care team – know who I can ask and get a handover from on the ward	• Can conduct assessment and devise management plans for communication problems post neurosurgery • Able to conduct swallow assessment in the ward setting • Confident in my communication skills with the colleagues I know on the ward	• Experienced in neurosurgical ward setting but limited experience in intensive care where patients are less stable • Lots of equipment I am unfamiliar with • I don't know the team or the routine, I'm worried about when it's the best time to go to the unit • Recent bereavement of grandparent I was close to and who recently had intensive care stay	• Like to feel in control and competent. • Concerned I will look inexperienced alongside experts • I feel I tend to work very slowly when I am uncertain and I am worried that I need to work quickly when I go to the unit
Platform for practice for neuro-intensive care uncertainty			

Figure 10.2 Illustrative platform for practice drawing retrospectively on uncertainty about working in intensive care

I find this approach concretely demonstrates the multiple and overlapping factors which contribute to a practice uncertainty. It can guide supervisor and supervisee to identify a promising place to focus as they start to work out how best to resolve the concern. I suggest this is much as we do clinically with complex problems, identifying the constituent parts and working methodically through an evidence-informed plan. The platform for practice also helps to identify strengths and the areas of practice where the supervisee may feel more secure. In my experience, a tendency to overlook this possibility as we focus on deficits misses opportunities to build on what is going well.

The platform for practice approach also acknowledges that things going on outside of practice can impact how secure the practitioner is feeling and that personal qualities, beliefs and behaviours can be important too. This is not to suggest that supervisors need to support all these dimensions. Indeed, supervisors need to be adept at recognising when a supervisee's concern lies outside of the supervisor's capability and to identify when supervision has crossed the boundary between formative and training, normative and fitness to practice, or restorative and counselling, for example. Breaking the concern down in terms of a platform for practice helps to clarify what might support effective navigation of the uncertainty and who is best placed to provide any necessary support including further training, joint working, in-practice supervision, psychological support and so on.

Supervision as a place to share and explore practice uncertainties: the place of an integrated model

In my intensive care example, it would be unlikely that one human, however skilful and experienced, could have assisted with every dimension of my uncertainty. I would have needed a combination of feeling safe to share my uncertainties and opportunities to develop my practice. This illustrates what I describe as the sanctuary and meta-practice functions of supervision. The sanctuary function offers space to share uncertainties safely, while meta-practice (a practice about practice) refers to exploring and identifying effective ways to resolve uncertainties or build on strengths. Importantly, resolving an uncertainty will sometimes mean eliminating it. At other times it involves being reassured that this is an inevitable uncertainty and working out how best to tolerate and navigate it. In my view, these sanctuary and meta-practice functions are not necessarily fulfilled by the same supervisor or as part of the same supervisory encounter. Indeed, supervision can be richer when we actively and collaboratively match the supervisor to the uncertainty.

As a small profession, SLTs do not always have the luxury of multiple supervisors or choice but I think we and other professions are sometimes blinkered. A mono-supervisory approach seems to squeeze too much under one supervision umbrella and expects too much of individual supervisors. One alternative (NHS 2020) proposes an integrated model combining a coordinating supervisor (we might call this a principal supervisor) with access to associate supervisors, matched to specific aspects of practitioner capability. In my neurosurgery example, my principal supervisor may have been a more senior SLT but perhaps more experienced in neurorehabilitation than in neurosurgery or intensive care. They may have been well-equipped to provide restorative supervision, support socio-professional or rehabilitation aspects of my practice. An associate supervisor or supervisors, not necessarily an SLT, could have offered valuable support for specific formative and normative aspects of my neurosurgical and intensive care practice. The key point here is about matching supervisor capability with the supervisee's uncertainty. We have wrestled with this a lot in multi-professional advanced practice. In healthcare we often default to uni-professional approaches which regard the supervisor as omni-capable when there is a rich multi-professional workforce well-positioned to supervise specific aspects of practice. I am not suggesting stepping outside of our registration to provide supervision for others without due consideration. I am suggesting there is value in adopting the approach registered professionals apply when deciding if a clinical activity sits within their clinical capability. In the context of supervision, this entails supervisors being satisfied that the aspect of practice they are supervising sits within their capability and registered scope of practice, regardless of whether the supervisee shares the supervisor's registration.

In my view, an integrated model offers the potential to combine private, reflective supervision with in-practice supervision to meet the breadth of supervisee needs. This will be most effective when practitioners feel able to share uncertainties safely with a supervisor who is both skilful in guiding and in recognising when the support required to navigate a practice concern lies outside of their professional/supervisory capability. Others have described enablers and barriers to effective supervision (Rothwell *et al.*, 2021). I would add that there are also behaviours which are useful for both supervisees and supervisors, and this is what I will discuss next.

Helpful behaviours and characteristics for supervision: being permeable.

In my research, I was first struck by colleagues' uncertainties. What grabbed me later was how practitioners varied in the extent to which they recognised uncertainties and sought to share these with others in their efforts to feel more secure in practice.

I noticed a cluster of behaviours which seem valuable (self-aware, aware of and for others, awareness-sharing, feedback-seeking, open to alternatives, critically aware, willing to change). I describe these as practitioner permeability (Figure 10.3). I use permeability to describe this cluster of behaviours but acknowledge some alignment with (Kelly, 1963) who wrote about permeable constructs.

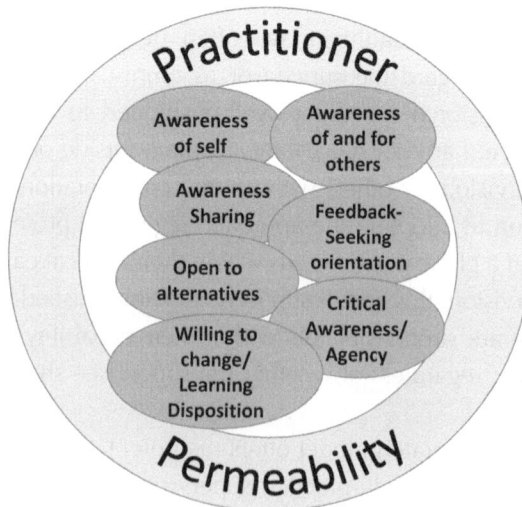

Figure 10.3 Dimensions of practitioner permeability
(Harding 2019, p. 145; 2023b)

Permeable practitioners recognise uncertainty and are willing to talk about and to explore ways to navigate and resolve uncertainties. Imagine that I am an experienced SLT working in a community team. Part of my role is supporting older people in residential homes. Most weeks, I do swallow safety assessments. I regard this as a secure aspect of my practice. I supervise less experienced colleagues who are developing dysphagia assessment competence. A couple of people I have assessed recently developed chest infections. This unsettles me. One became very poorly. I start questioning my dysphagia competence. I have some uncertainty about my practice because I am *self-aware*. I am worried about the well-being of the people I assessed but also concerned about what others might be thinking too: the staff in the home, family of the people who fell ill, my colleagues, peers and supervisees. These are instances of my *awareness of and for others*. This self-awareness and awareness of and for others might make me more vigilant in future assessments or prompt me to access some refresher training. For a greater chance of success in resolving my uncertainty it helps if I am willing to share it; *awareness-sharing*. This may be with a trusted colleague in the office, in the car between visits or with a designated supervisor. Sometimes, awareness-sharing prompts a lightbulb moment which is enough to resolve the concern. I might decide to review whether the advice I had provided was followed as intended, how family and friends had been advised and so on. This might reassure me about my knowledge and skills but nudge me to look at the ways in which I hand over findings and recommendations. Of course, we do not always have lightbulb moments without also having some feedback. So, I should be actively *feedback-seeking* too, especially in an instance like this where there is a possible clinical risk. This means being willing to hear what my supervisor or another colleague thinks, considering their views and remaining open to the idea that I might receive uncomfortable, unexpected or previously unconsidered feedback and guidance. In other words, to make use of feedback I will need to be *open to alternatives*. For example, it might not have occurred to me to tighten up my handover until my supervisor suggests it. We might explore other alternatives too like refresher training or some shadowing and joint working with the supervisor. Ideally, together we will *critically appraise* the options for resolving my uncertainty to decide which will help me feel professionally safe and, importantly, that public safety is maintained. Not always, but in some instances, maintaining professional and public safety will necessitate changes to my current practices and so, the final part of the permeability cluster is a *willingness to change* and to maintain a career-long *learning disposition*.

Being permeable is not just helpful to the supervisee but also for supervisors. Table 10.2 provides some indicators of the dimensions of permeability for both supervisees and supervisors.

Table 10.2 Indicative supervisee and supervisor dimensions of permeability

Dimensions of practitioner permeability	Role	
	Supervisee	Supervisor
Self-aware	Recognises own uncertainties.	Recognises own position and experience. Recognises own practice uncertainties. Models self-awareness in practice.
Aware of and for others	Recognises implications for practice and safety: Public Colleagues	Uses own position and experience thoughtfully for supervisee, colleague and public benefit. Maintains a focus on professional and public safety.
Awareness sharing	Shares uncertainties with others.	Shares concerns and celebrates successes with supervisee.
Feedback seeking	Welcomes and considers feedback from others.	Welcomes feedback about self as a supervisor and educator.
Open to alternatives	Is open to other ways of doing and learning.	Explores alternative ways of doing and learning, recognising that other ways may be safe.
Critically aware	Weighs up what works and will be safe.	Weighs up what works and will be safe.
Willing to change/learn	Is willing to implement changes in practice.	Continues to engage in own professional development across the pillars of practice. Has appraisal objectives specific to supervisor development.

Permeable supervisors recognise their own limitations and the place of supervision in the context of a variety of options which will maximise practitioner and public safety. There will be times when the resolution of a supervisee's uncertainty lies outside of the one-to-one supervision encounter. Indeed, in my research I heard how it was unhelpful when a supervisor was rigid and inflexible, expecting the supervisee to do things exactly the way the supervisor preferred. Permeable supervisors do not seek to craft their supervisees as clones. They recognise a spectrum of safe practice and apply critical awareness to assess practitioner safety as part of their duty of care in keeping both their supervisee and the public safe. Permeable supervisors also maintain a career-long learning disposition, across the pillars of practice, acting as a role model for their supervisees.

It is not the case that some practitioners are tuned into uncertainties and others not. An individual can vary day by day and from one encounter to another. There are times in practice when we are more impermeable, when, even in the context of some uncertainty, we decide to stick with our position. For example, we might feel it is premature to discharge someone home and advocate to extend the admission when colleagues feel this is unnecessary. At other times we are more porous, looking for reassurance that we are doing what is expected, for example when we join a new rotation or encounter an unfamiliar diagnosis. We will recognise our own and colleagues' tendencies to be more or less permeable. There are those we perceive are set in their ways and determined to continue as they have always done, even when those ways do not seem to serve them very well and others who seem more porous, seeking yet more training, support and guidance. Being permeable enough to navigate practice successfully requires the practitioner to stay alert to these variations, judging when to share uncertainties and what feedback or alternatives to apply to practice. The emphasis on evidence-based practice has perhaps led us to regard uncertainty as a marker for risk, but the permeable practitioner's learning disposition means uncertainty is also recognised as a prompt to learn and to apply that learning to mitigate risk. Permeability, along with our uncertainties, will be dynamic and fluctuating. It may reassure the reader that although I can see how helpful these behaviours are, I am not always a beacon of permeability and I remain very much a work in progress. Reflecting on one's permeability, either as supervisor or supervisee, can be valuable and for those who wish to do so with some structure, permeability self-assessment questions can be helpful (Harding, 2023b).

Thawed, permeable and persuaded

Through my work across healthcare I have warmed to supervision. It provides vital opportunities to share and explore inevitable practice uncertainties. When there are conditions of trust and collaboration between supervisor and supervisee, supervision provides an opportunity to regard uncertainties as a prompt to learn, be that about self and others or about technical knowledge and skills. Supervision is optimised when both supervisor and supervisee are permeable. Permeable supervision focuses on practice uncertainties which both supervisor and supervisee care about and care to resolve. While some dimensions of a practice concern may relate to personal factors, the supervisor is focused on the implications for practice; not passing personal judgment but recognising a duty of care to the supervisee to ensure they are the safest practitioner possible. When both supervisee and supervisor are permeable, they are motivated not only by professional safety but by their duty of care to the public.

This idea that supervision is the cornerstone of professional and public safety has been recognised long before my need to feel more persuaded. For those wiser sooner than me, this chapter may have been an irritating read. However, for much of the health system the supervision awakening has been slow. Earlier I shared concerns that more insights were needed if employers and decision-makers were to appreciate the value of supervision and recognise it as something other than a drain on productivity. There are signs that a supervision spring is beginning to bloom and there is much to thank Kirkup (2015) for in this regard. His recommendation that the regulatory and professional aspects of supervision should be separated so that employers take responsibility for workplace supervision has prompted health providers to take their responsibilities seriously (Health and Social Care Act 2008(Regulated Activities) 2014, Regulations 12 and 18). The independent regulator of health and care in England, the Care Quality Commission (CQC, 2023) directs employers to these legal responsibilities, as do NHS Employers (2022). For supervision to flourish and for professionals and the public to feel and be safe will take more than these governance sticks. Supervision is an important, regular point of sanctuary and meta-practice. We cannot expect that all our uncertainties will be eliminated through supervision but it does provide an opportunity to identify a range of options for navigating and resolving uncertainty, including building on secure practice.

I am persuaded that we are justified in protecting time for supervision in and on practice as a vital aspect of professional and public safety. However, we must continue to invest in the development of supervisor capability, to capture the return on investment in this development in terms of safety, quality and productivity, to be permeable and to remain open to the learning possibilities which accompany our inevitable, career-long, practice uncertainties.

References

Appleby, A., Galea, A. and Murray, R. (2014) The NHS productivity challenge: experience from the front line. Kings Fund. Available online at: https://www.kingsfund.org.uk/sites/default/files/field/field_publication_file/the-nhs-productivity-challenge-kingsfund-may14.pdf [Last accessed: 01.07.23].

Clouder, L. and Sellars, J. (2004) Reflective practice and clinical supervision: an interprofessional perspective. *Journal of Advanced Nursing*, 46(3), 262–269.

CQC (2023) Guidance for providers. Available online at: www.cqc.org.uk/guidance [Last accessed: 04.07.23].

Dall'Alba, G. (2009) Learning professional ways of being: Ambiguities of becoming. *Educational Philosophy and Theory*, 41(1), 34–45.

Dall'Alba, G. and Barnacle, R. (2015) Exploring knowing/being through discordant professional practice. *Educational Philosophy and Theory*, 47(13–14), 1452–1464.

Duchscher, J. E. B. (2009) Transition shock: The initial stake of role adaptation for newly graduated Registered Nurses. *Journal of Advanced Nursing* 65(5), 1103–1113

Eraut, M. (1994) *Developing Professional Knowledge and Competence*. London: Routledge.

Fox, R. (1957) Training for uncertainty. In R. K. Merton, G. Reader and P. L. Kendall (eds) *The Student Physician*. Cambridge: Harvard University Press.

Gilbert, T. (2001) Reflective practice and clinical supervision: meticulous rituals of the confessional. *Journal of Advanced Nursing*, 36, 199–205

Harding, D. (2019) Practitioner permeability and the resolution of practice uncertainties: a grounded theoretical perspective of supervision for allied health professionals. PhD thesis, St George's, University of London. Available online: https://eprints.kingston.ac.uk/43854/6/Harding-D-43854.pdf

Harding, D. (2023a) Working with the idea of a platform for practice. Available online at: https://thepermeablepractitioner.com/ideas-and-resources/working-with-the-idea-of-a-platform-for-practice/ [Last accessed: 04.07.23].

Harding, D. (2023b) Working with the idea of practitioner permeability. Available online at: https://thepermeablepractitioner.com/ideas-and-resources/working-with-the-idea-of-practitioner-permeability/ [Last accessed: 04.07.23].

HCPC (2023) Standards of proficiency for practice. Available online at: www. hcpc-uk.org/standards/standards-of-proficiency/ [Last accessed: 03.07.2023].

Health and Social Care Act (2008) Regulated Activities (2014) Available online at: www.legislation.gov.uk/ukdsi/2014/9780111117613/contents [Last accessed: 04.07.23].

Kelly, G. (1963) *A Theory of Personality: The Psychology of Personal Constructs.* New York: Norton

Kirkup, B. (2015) The report of the Morecambe Bay investigation. London: The Stationery Office. Available online at: https://assets.publishing.service.gov.uk/government/uploads/system/uploads/attachment_data/file/408480/47487_MBI_Accessible_v0.1.pdf [Last accessed: 04.07.23].

Lynch, L., Happell, B. and Sharrock, J. (2008). Clinical supervision: an exploration of its origins and definitions. *International Journal of Psychiatric Nursing Research,* 13(2).

NHS (2020) Workplace supervision for advanced clinical practice: An integrated multiprofessional approach for practitioner development. Available online at: https://advanced-practice.hee.nhs.uk/workplace-supervision-for-advanced-clinical-practice-2/ [Last accessed: 04.07.23].

NHS Employers (2022) Clinical Supervision Models for Registered Professionals. Available online at: www.nhsemployers.org/articles/clinical-supervision-models-registered-professionals [Last accessed: 04.07.23].

Proctor, B. (2008) *Group Supervision: A Guide to Creative Practice,* 2nd edn. London: Sage

Revans, R. (2011) *ABC of Action Learning.* Farnham: Gower

Rolfe, G. (2011) Reflection-in-action. In G. Rolfe, M. Jasper and D. Freshwater (eds) *Critical Reflection in Practice; Generating Knowledge for Care,* 2nd edn. London: Macmillan International.

Rolfe, G. and Gardener, L. (2006) 'Do not ask who I am . . .' Confession, emancipation and (self)-management through reflection. *Journal of Nursing Management,* 14, 593–600.

Rothwell, C., Kehoe, A., Farook, S. F. and Illing, J. (2021) Enablers and barriers to effective clinical supervision in the workplace: a rapid evidence review. *BMJ Open,* 11, e052929. doi:10.1136/bmjopen-2021-052929

Schön, D. A. (1983) *The Reflective Practitioner: How Professionals Think in Action.* New York: Basic Books.

Webster-Wright, A. (2010) *Authentic Professional Learning: Making a Difference Through Learning at Work.* London: Springer.

11

Must it Always Be Within, or Could it Be Outside?
Constructions of Supervision Outside Your Own Profession

Fran Brander and Gavin Newby

Supervision is one of the cornerstones of clinical governance throughout the UK health sector. UK Professional bodies and the Health and Care Professions Council (HCPC) rightly set out supervisory standards and expectations of behaviour. In the main, supervision is most often construed as a within profession group activity, essentially looking after your own. Whilst supervision from your own professional grouping has many advantages, we, Fran Brander (a National Health Service (NHS) Consultant Physiotherapist) and Gavin Newby (a Consultant Clinical Neuropsychologist in private practice) argue in this chapter that receiving supervision from outside your profession is not only a sensible and practical way of ensuring everyone has access to supervision but can very much be a positive and growing experience. The insights of other professions and individuals can only expand perspectives and frames.

Our aim is to produce a readable and accessible chapter on the benefits of supervision from another profession. We have tried not to assume any particular specialist or theoretical knowledge. We have, however, made some references to Personal Construct Psychology (PCP). This is because PCP offers a way of noticing words, phrases or feelings that resonate for us and allows exploration of what they might mean. PCP calls these concepts 'constructs', words or phrases loaded with meaning and which predict a person's approach and action to a situation (Fransella and Dalton, 2000). The word 'supervision' is a good example – what it means for you as a reader will have origins in your experience of supervision in the past and may be very different from ours (whose will be different from each other's) and be very individual to you.

DOI: 10.4324/9781003301141-11

> **Reflective point**
>
> It certainly has not been lost on us that there are many obvious inter-personal parallels about us being two people from different profes-sional backgrounds collaborating on a chapter about supervision from outside our professions. We have continually reflected on this as we wrote the chapter and think that it has helped us appreciate the benefits of outside supervision working all the more.

Supervision comes in many guises and forms. Supervision has many different meanings depending on your setting, what is available and what looks and feels like supervision. Many people have written excellent articles and chapters on supervision and its 'gears' (which range from education to counselling to coaching and managing to name a few) and functions (rang-ing from welfare monitoring to skills acquisition to professional safeguard-ing). There are many forms from individual to group and now of course to remote. Interested readers can easily tap into readable summaries written by Joyce Scaife (2019).

We thought that it would be helpful here to make clear what the con-struct of 'supervision' might not be. Anybody working in any kind of clinical setting will have experienced more conversational and informal interactions with colleagues that they work with, whether within your pro-fession or outside. These can range from an extended water cooler moment to discussions over lunch (e.g., see Newby, Bichard, Campbell, Odiyoor, & Pinder, 2017) to 'can we discuss this over a coffee or a pint'. These inter-actions are, of course, really important and valuable. We would not seek to downplay or disregard them but would see them as professional col-league support rather than supervision. In our view, professional support is no adequate replacement for supervision. Broadly speaking, in most UK healthcare settings, supervision tends to be provided in clinical and mana-gerial forms. Probably the most common type of supervision in the NHS is managerial – supervision provided by someone senior to you and usually within your profession. Much of the content of this supervision will be focused on organisational tasks, such as how well you are meeting service or departmental targets, managing caseloads etc. Professional supervision, by contrast, is focused on helping the supervisee understand or make sense of a clinical problem and develop ideas and solutions to get round it (e.g. understanding why someone may not be engaging and thinking about ways of getting them back on board).

In this chapter we talk about our own respective experiences of professional supervision from, and with, somebody from a different profession. In fact, we celebrate its virtues. We have some experiences and views which are similar and some which are contrasting. So, in order to help you understand what we both agree on and how we see things as individuals, we have decided to write this chapter in the first person as 'we' when we speak as the both of us. But also we use 'I' when referring to only one of our voices and assign whose voice it is (e.g., **Fran writes**:).

Our supervision histories and their influence on this chapter

We both have 30 years' experience in our respective fields, predominantly in neurosciences. Supervision has always been a key element in our learning and development, and we have experienced and provided various types of supervision. We are able to extoll the virtues of supervision from outside our professions because we have both participated in supervision with a practitioner who is a PCP Counsellor and Speech and Language Therapist who also works in neurosciences. For the purpose of this chapter we will refer to this supervisor as our/my *outside* supervisor. In our opinion this has been a particularly open and freeing experience precisely because this practitioner is neither a Neuropsychologist nor a Physiotherapist. Although we refer throughout this chapter to our specific experiences of being in supervision with our outside supervisor, these are only our examples. We hope the reader will be able to extract the important components that are relevant to them from our experiences. In addition, as we discuss later, the reader's choice is no longer limited to who you can meet in person, with the recent advent of widespread tele-conferencing, there are numerous excellent supervisors with a range of professional backgrounds who you will be able to access.

Fran writes: I had known my outside supervisor for many years and was encouraged to ask her to be my supervisor by a colleague who had experienced supervision with her and thought we would work well together.

137

I had not considered how supervision by someone in another profession would differ from previous experiences, although I was interested in receiving supervision from someone outside my workplace. However, I have benefitted from both her experience, the fact that she heralds from a different discipline and in addition that she is external to my organisation. Physiotherapy is a practical profession and previous supervision had reflected that and always been solution-focussed. Supervision with my outside supervisor is more reflective. She does not have first-hand knowledge of my work processes, colleagues and their characteristics, or of specific background situations. She is objective, helping me to explore all aspects of any given situation, including my feelings and emotional response to them. She allows me to explore resolutions that I may or may not be comfortable with, and ultimately enables me to choose the response that feels most authentic to me. Being supervised by someone without a background in physiotherapy really works for me for several reasons. We have an excellent relationship based on mutual trust and respect, the approach is reflective and exploratory rather than solution-focussed and together we explore how I might best respond to people and situations, ensuring I remain true to myself. I feel as though I have grown in terms of my emotional intelligence, rather than responding with knee-jerk reactions that ultimately may not be helpful.

Gavin writes: In contrast to Fran I have been fortunate enough to have supervision from several practitioners outside my profession including a consultant psychiatrist who was working with older adults in the same team as me and, more recently, our outside supervisor. Their experience just oozes out of them. I have particularly valued their interpersonal warmth, openness, humour and flexibility. Both of them have a very intuitive ability to step equally into my shoes and those involved in any case or situation being discussed. These two practitioners have worked with a vast range of clients, families and situations in their own contexts and can therefore bring a sage viewpoint to any dilemma. The psychiatrist gave me some excellent psychodynamic supervision that has had career-long impacts, particularly in providing me with an appreciation of the ideas of reverie and holding in mind within the works of Melanie Klein and Wilfred Bion (Waddell, 1998). This helps me to this day appreciate the power of the therapeutic relationship and the importance of a deeper, mostly non-verbal process that can happen in productive and working therapeutic relationships. This is where one can develop a sense of what the other might be thinking and can anticipate issues and thoughts. This is the reverie that Klein discusses where the client feels safe, secure, and held. The psychiatrist taught me how impactful it is for clients to know that we hold them in mind and consider their well-being outside of our sessions (Newby, 2013).

Gavin continues: When I left the NHS in 2016, I understood my professional obligation to source and receive regular supervision. I saw this as an opportunity to seek a supervisor who would not only fulfil an obligation but also challenge and expand my reflective practice. I have been supervised by my outside supervisor on a six-weekly basis since that time. It was a conscious decision to choose her, having been impressed by her clinical reflectiveness and knowledge when completing two PCP courses with her. Whilst warm and open I knew she would not hesitate to challenge, which has been the case. I have particularly valued the practicality of her suggestions and willingness to help me operationalise my wonderings across a wide range of topics. PCP is often notoriously written in a hard-to-understand way, and she has become my pathfinder. There is a focus on PCP as you would expect but also a flexibility to go with the flow – I love that. On reflection, I wonder if the key constructs for me in a supervisor are around openness, trust, and oscillating between freedom and safe containment when it is needed.

The ingredients of accessing supervision from outside your profession

In this section we discuss the key ingredients we feel are helpful for successful supervision from outside your profession:

a. Context and choice

What we bring to a supervisory relationship, what is expected and what the eventual perceived product may be, can be dependent on what the organisational context is. For example, in the NHS a supervisor is assigned to a practitioner on the basis of availability, greater experience, seniority or being your manager rather than being a fit to your needs. Whether or not you have any choice in who supervises you is important, but is it a game changer?

Gavin writes: In my experience, the supervisors assigned to me have been dependent on my seniority, the availability of supervision, the organisational trends of my workplace and funding available for any external supervision.

When I worked in the NHS, choice was initially limited to the more senior psychologist who was available, and typically, my manager. I had some excellent supervision but had no choice about who they were and whether they came from within or outside my profession. That said, early on in my career, the on-the-job learning from more experienced psychologists and managers taught me a great deal about being a psychologist and understanding the NHS. I also experienced that the availability of supervision was often determined by organisational trends within the NHS. An example of this was going from a psychology departmental model towards psychologists being scattered across various different teams. This meant a mixed model of some case-related supervision from a psychologist but managerial supervision (covering such as caseload numbers and type of cases) from an outside profession manager. Again, some excellent supervision occurred but there was often a tension created between, for example, the organisational pressure to see more referred clients and to discharge someone to make space, before I felt I had addressed all their needs. As I progressed to consultant grade and became the 'experienced neuropsychologist', greater choice was on the agenda but only in the form of being a neuropsychologist of a similar or greater experience. My NHS Trust (UK healthcare service provider) did, however, accept that I could source supervision from outside that organisation. I was able to access excellent within-profession supervision with the head of a geographically nearby neuropsychology service. I suspect others may have been less privileged with funding. Currently I work entirely privately and manage my own work. As a result I have been free to choose a supervisor irrespective of profession. The frame of requiring a supervisor to satisfy professional and HCPC reasons of course remains.

Fran writes: The managerial supervision I receive from my Physiotherapy manager, whilst being very supportive, is inevitably influenced by the needs of the NHS Trust, the service and the teams that I am directly responsible for. Conversely, supervision from my outside supervisor is largely driven by my personal and professional needs, whatever they may be at the time. Having a supervisor from a different profession allows me the freedom to be more self-focussed regarding what I want to bring to supervision that day, and we can fully explore all nuances of my situation, others' reactions or behaviours and my response or behaviour consequently. I need to be clear what I want from outside supervision and whether my potential supervisor can meet that, in terms of their approach and the more personal aspects of the relationship (mutual respect, openness and willingness on both sides to explore alternative solutions). As stated before, I want to acknowledge that when choosing an outside supervisor I also recognise the value of that person being from an external service, organisation or business. This means that they will not be aware of or caught up in specific personnel or politics which can be a huge advantage.

b. Levelling the relationship

We would both agree that a successful supervision experience from outside your profession is likely to be underlain by both participants consciously sharing the core value of equity. There are always going to be pupil-teacher moments, such as when the supervisor is describing a concept or technique you have not previously come across. This has its place of course, but the relationship is unlikely to remain positive if it stays stuck in that 'teaching' mode. The supervisory relationship needs to be flexible and interchangeable. Similarly, an outside supervisory relationship that did not clarify initial stances, constructs and dynamics would stay stuck in that teacher-pupil construction, possibly making it difficult to truly challenge and let different perspectives emerge.

Reflective point

We have been aware of how the process of writing this chapter together parallels this important supervisory dynamic. The content of our initial meetings was dominated by confirming our professional experiences, years in the job and current working contexts; 'checking each other out' as it were. Although this contact established a mutual credibility, it also highlighted some differences that felt uncomfortable. For example, we noticed marked differences in the extent to which we had published articles and chapters about our work. In subsequent contact, we both worked hard to confirm that we have equally important things to share and can learn from each other.

Fran writes: Prior to working with my outside supervisor, I received and offered within profession (professional and managerial) supervision which followed a routine format (e.g. a standardised proforma, an exchange of information and an advice/solution focussed style). Having chosen an outside supervisor, it came as a bit of a shock when she suggested at our first meeting that we might agree a 'contract' – a flexible agreement detailing the ways in which we could work together, as two 'experts' in the room and foregrounding how I as the supervisee might like to use the space. This was a first and an eye opener for me. She saw supervision as a mutual process that needed to work for both supervisee and supervisor. We both have responsibility for effective supervision and on reflection I think that is one of the reasons why it works so well. To be a good fit it is a two-way relationship; a supervisor cannot supervise me effectively if I am not willing or able to participate fully, openly and honestly and likewise the same needs to be the case for the supervisor. We believe that all supervision should include a contract or agreement, but we both suspect that this is often not the case.

c. Celebrating difference

There can definitely be advantages to having an outside supervisor. For both of us, it is enlightening having a supervisor who does not share all our background and experiences. They can look at situations with a new perspective, take more chances, be less constrained by a professional view or prejudice and there is no such thing as the 'departmental view'. Outside supervision feels fresh rather than alien and deeper questioning through naivety allows exploration of the wider context.

Fran writes: I have learnt a lot about how my whole profession is perceived from someone of another profession. For example, physiotherapy is one of the largest Allied Health Professions (AHP). Therefore, in terms of influence, physiotherapy may have a louder voice just by sheer numbers. I had never considered this until it was pointed out and reflected on in supervision, nor the impact therefore that this might have on those I work with from other professions. Supervision from a different professional background can heighten our self-awareness as an individual and facilitate reflection in terms of our professional identity.

We both feel that an outside supervisor needs, of course, to share something with you (e.g. working therapeutically with clients or understanding something of your work context). However, whilst having familiarity is a helpful glue for the supervisory relationship, a downside of familiarity can be limits to seeing issues and solutions with fresh eyes. In our experience, not being of the same profession makes it more possible to walk in the other person's shoes with less fear. Discussions and possible steps to a solution are more likely to be novel.

d. Be clear what you are looking for

Everyone can learn from their supervision experiences whether good or bad, and those experiences will guide how you feel about the supervision you are receiving at this time and whether it does or does not quite fit the bill. Consequently your constructs around supervision will influence whether you accept what you are receiving or whether you proactively seek out a new relationship. When you decide you need a change in your supervision arrangements, we suggest you take the chance to reflect on what has or has not worked for you before. This might help you to widen your lens to include seeking a supervisor from outside your profession. Perhaps you are looking to: freshen up your work motivation, give you new perspectives, allow you more dedicated time for reflection, have the freedom to explore different approaches? Entering into a new relationship, particularly with an outside supervisor, can be a golden opportunity to articulate your different hopes and aspirations for what you want to use that supervision space for.

e. The value of teleconferencing

COVID and lockdowns brought teleconferencing to the fore, for therapy sessions, meetings and also for supervision. We imagine that some of your supervisory relationships have remained online, long after COVID has receded. You might even be considering or already accessing supervision from a colleague who lives in a different country.

Gavin writes: Teleconferencing is impossible to ignore given the COVID pandemic, it has found a permanent place in the world of supervision. It can certainly work, in my experience, as my outside supervisor and I both live in different parts of the UK. It is visual, it has sound, it is live. It can be a very effective therapeutic and supervisory medium. Maybe a totally teleconferenced relationship might lack something? I had met my outside supervisor in real life before setting up the relationship and think it helps to meet at least once in the flesh. Poor internet connection, time lapses, difficulties logging in, are issues that I have had to face over the last few years. The strength of our relationship minimised any impact this may have had on my supervision sessions, but I have no doubt they would have had more of an impact had we not already established at least some in person rapport. In my therapeutic work I have a provisional idea of a dose effect; essentially actual face-face meetings are needed at some point whether to start it all off or to refresh an ongoing relationship.

f. Making sure supervision reflects your changing needs over time

Like any relationship, what you need from supervision will evolve and change as you gain experience or change context.[1] Without sounding too trite, supervision, just like everything else in life, is a journey. What might be right at the beginning of your career (more a pupil-teacher dynamic) may not be as appropriate for you as you gain experience. Early on something akin to an apprenticeship-type relationship may be appropriate as the more experienced practitioner demonstrates and teaches particular skills. The newly qualified therapist may hang on every word of the supervisor but as the supervisee gains more experience, they will have a broader knowledge base to draw on, developing more of their own ideas and feeling able to challenge. As therapists become experienced, they may want to reflect on themes arising across clients and situations rather than seek advice about a specific situation.

We would be surprised to hear that a newly qualified AHP was receiving supervision from someone outside their profession. But as the very nature of our roles is interdisciplinary, why should a new graduate not receive *both* within and outside supervision? The key here is ensuring that your own profession and HCPC guidance is adhered to. We believe that you need within discipline supervision as the main supervision to ensure you gain the fundamental knowledge but if you were to receive supervision from outside in addition might that be the icing on the cake?

g. It is not one relationship at the expense of all others

During supervision sessions with our outside supervisor we have both spoken about the advantages of practitioners seeking a 'smorgasbord' of supervisory experiences. What works well for someone could be a portfolio of people, places, contexts, groups that, combined, meet all your needs.

Fran writes: I have professional supervision with my outside supervisor, managerial supervision with my physiotherapy manager, as well as professional support from my colleagues at work (whatever their seniority or profession). Consequently, all my needs are addressed. However, it is important that I regularly review the range of sources of supervision and support I am receiving, in case I need to alter the balance at any time.

Our five key considerations

Supervision is a very personal phenomenon based on a human relationship. What we summarise below is not a prescription but will hopefully help you consider the benefits of seeking supervision from outside your profession:

1. Why?

If you are thinking about supervision from another profession, please listen to yourself! Ask yourself some questions. For example is it because you have got into a rut, feel too comfortable, not comfortable enough, have seen or heard about someone from another profession who could shake you out of that rut? Maybe you have found some more headspace recently to want to push the edges of your thinking? Is there something constraining about your current practice and experience of supervision. Maybe you feel that you are not always open to new ideas?

More importantly we would strongly advocate that there comes a time in your career when the question should be 'why wouldn't you seek supervision from outside your profession?' Particularly if you have not experienced different styles and approaches to supervision. Trying something new will broaden your horizons and enable greater growth, both personally and professionally as supervisee and supervisor. You cannot know what is possible until you have explored multiple avenues and experiences.

2. Who?

Look out for somebody who might share some of your core values and with whom you might have equality. Find someone you believe has credibility which can, in turn, develop into a positive relationship. Ideally, you may have had some interpersonal experience of the potential outside supervisor in another context, maybe having met them at a conference, attended a course run by them or talked with them at a meeting. Having some sort of pre-existing experience and sense of connection with your potential outside supervisor can put the prospect of being supervised by them in a positive frame from the outset. You may already have felt that you could work with them, had positive experiences of sharing clients and can imagine a productive supervisory relationship. However this is not to say that you could not have a very successful supervisory relationship with someone whom you only know by reputation or from their writing. Perhaps more importantly, consider organising an introductory session and making sure that you regularly review how it is going. If it works, great, if not, can you both adapt to feedback? Not every relationship can work, and it may be that you need to try more than one supervisor before finding the right fit.

3. What?

The exact form of outside supervision may depend on multiple factors such as the time available, funding and organisational view. It may not be the only supervision you have; you might be accessing different types of supervision for different reasons. It may only be for a short time or for a few sessions. You do not have to put all your eggs in one basket at the expense of anything else that your setting and context has to offer. You might be able to have the best of both worlds: supervision within and outside. Remember supervision can be in a variety of forms; individual from someone more experienced is the most familiar but peer supervision and group supervision can also be excellent (see other chapters in this book for a discussion of both).

4. When?

In our opinion, you are more likely to seek outside supervision at a more experienced time of your career, after the foundations of your job role (as imbibed from a more senior colleague within your profession) have been fully explored and when you are ready to expand your possibilities. Also, in our experience outside supervision is more likely to be supported when you are more senior. That said, even if you are a senior practitioner within your organisation it can be a significant challenge to get the backing of managers for the time and funding to obtain supervision outside your profession. You may have to sell the benefits of such supervision with a sceptical and budget-orientated funder. A creative approach can pay dividends such as being prepared to see that supervisor outside of the working day, offering some teaching in exchange or taking up opportunities to earn additional funds for your organisation or to self-fund.

For those of you early in your career, supervision from within your own profession is vital. But we believe that with some creativity it is possible to have valuable and relevant conversations with other disciplines in your MDT as part of professional support. For example, you could ask the Occupational Therapist (OT) to discuss how they formulate the complexity of a client's problems from their professional perspective, or you could spend a nursing shift observing how they work with your client. These relationships can gradually build to a point where later in your career you understand the value of seeking supervision from a profession that is outside your own.

5. How?

That is up to you! You will need to be creative, opportunistic and self-motivated. Perhaps discuss this with your current supervisor. Continue to reflect on the fit of your supervisory experiences. Keep your supervisory antennae on. Touch base with the practitioners you meet in professional networks, conferences and the like. Keep experimenting with the format and providers of supervision.

Concluding thoughts

In essence, we are both ardent supporters of professional supervision with someone outside our own profession. Of course, context is everything and supervision from wherever it is sourced can easily feel uncomfortable if the context is one where you are being forced, judged or monitored. Agreeing shared goals and creating a collaborative negotiated contract to support the supervision relationship is key. Within this framework of outside supervision, the supervisor and supervisee can unlock exciting new perspectives, enabling freedom to explore the wider context. This in turn can lead to novel discussions, approaches & solutions, resulting in greater growth and self-awareness, both personally and professionally.

Note

1 We do acknowledge that many readers may not be in a position to exercise a great deal of choice about their supervisor. However, even if being able to choose someone from outside your profession feels impossible, you may well be able to mould your supervisory relationship to reflect what you need.

References

Fransella, F. & Dalton, P. (2000) *Personal Constructs in Action*, 2nd edn. Sage: London.

Newby, G. (2013) Introduction: Understanding how to work with acquired brain injury or how to be or not to be: that is the crucial question in brain injury in: G. Newby, R. Coetzer, A. Daisley & S. Weatherhead (Eds.) (2013) *Practical Neuropsychological Rehabilitation in Acquired Brain Injury: A Guide for Working Clinicians*. London: Karnac Books.

Newby, G., Bichard, H., Campbell, N., Odiyoor, M. & Pinder, C. (2017) Reclaiming the lost art of lunch. *BMJ Blog*. Available online at: http://blogs.bmj.com/bmj/2017/05/02/gavin-newby-reclaiming-the-lost-art-of-lunch/ [Accessed 29 January, 2022].

Scaife, J. (2019) *Supervision in Clinical Practice. A Practitioner's Guide*, 3rd edn. Hove, Bruner-Routledge.

Waddell, M. (1998) *Inside Lives: Psychoanalysis and the Growth of the Personality*. London: Duckworth.

12

Developing a Multi-Disciplinary Allied Health Professional Supervision Strategy
A Case Study

Lucie Rochfort

This chapter sets out a project undertaken in an acute United Kingdom National Health Service (NHS) hospital organisation (a hospital Trust), to review and refresh clinical supervision across the therapy professions. The project was initiated through engagement in multi-professional supervision training commissioned by the Head of Therapies. The training generated discussion and debate about the range of perspectives and variety of methods and approaches to clinical supervision across the different teams and professions in Therapy Services and while some particularly good practice was noted, scope for more work was also identified. A project was carried out to develop a clinical supervision resource pack with guidance, training, templates, and other resources with the goal to promote high-quality supervision and enhance the supervision experience. This, in turn, would support staff wellbeing and ensure safe and high-quality clinical practice. This chapter will describe the project, from the review of existing supervision arrangements to the development and implementation of the resource pack. Perceived benefits and challenges relating to the project are shared. This includes the unanticipated interruptions of the Covid-19 pandemic, demonstrating that new and creative ways of working and approaching clinical supervision are very possible and can be implemented at short notice. The chapter concludes that navigating these challenges has highlighted the need to keep clinical supervision at the forefront of people's minds and to recognise the importance of supervision for staff wellbeing and as a safe space to explore clinical practice.

It is important to note that the term 'clinical supervision' is used throughout this chapter. This is because it was the term most widely used and

DOI: 10.4324/9781003301141-12

understood amongst the different professions within the department where this project took place. The Royal College of Speech and Language Therapists Information on Supervision (RCSLT, 2017) guidance refers to this as professional supervision and reports it can sometimes also be known as personal or practice supervision. However, for the purpose of consistency and clarity within the project the term clinical supervision was used.

Background

I am a speech and language therapist (SLT) by profession and have always been aware of the need for regular, good quality supervision for myself and my colleagues to enable us to provide high-quality care, be safe and effective and to support our wellbeing. The regulator of health and care professions in the UK, the Health and Care Professions Council's (HCPC), standards of proficiency for speech and language therapists state that in order to 'be able to practise as an autonomous professional, exercising their own professional judgement' we must 'understand the need for active participation in training, supervision and mentoring' (HCPC, 2023, pp. 8–9). Our professional body, the Royal College of Speech and Language Therapists (RCSLT) Information on Supervision (2017) document contains guidance, along with recommendations regarding what supervision is and at what frequency it should be happening. Despite this, my own experience of supervision over my career has been extremely variable. At its best it provides an invaluable opportunity to reflect on professional practice, at its worst it is a redundant, tick box exercise.

More recently, as a service manager in an acute hospital, I have become even more aware of the value of having effective supervision systems. Managing multi-professional teams of SLTs, dietitians, occupational therapists and physiotherapists gave me unique insight into how the different professions approach supervision with their diverse views and practices. As a manager, it was evident that clinical supervision is not just for individual professional development and wellbeing but an essential way to ensure the staff within my services were supported to deliver effective, evidence-based care to a high standard. In this position I had the privilege of overseeing the development of a clinical supervision resource pack by a multi-professional working group. This chapter describes the process the working group went through in developing and sharing the resource pack, as well as the benefits

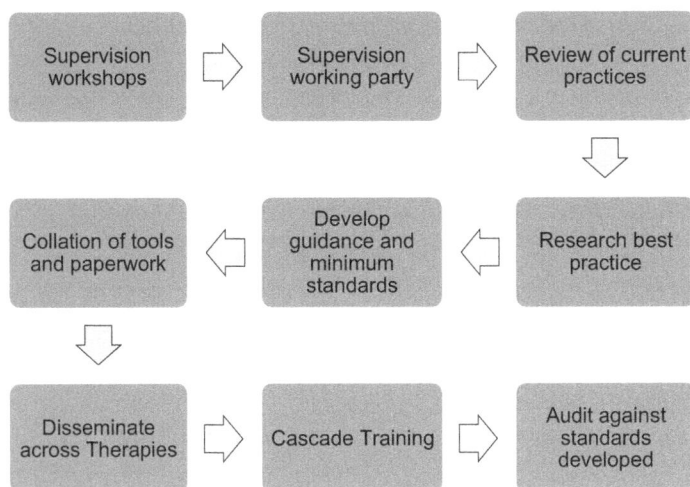

Figure 12.1 Process of supervision strategy development

and challenges we had along the way. The stages of supervision strategy development we engaged in are summarised in Figure 12.1 and are subsequently discussed in further detail.

Towards the end of 2018, the Head of Therapies commissioned supervision workshops facilitated by a university-based academic. This was attended by a group of SLTs, dietitians, physiotherapists and occupational therapists from various different clinical areas, all working at specialist or team lead level and with an interest in clinical supervision. The workshops covered the themes of:

- What do we think supervision is?
- Evidence-base and literature which informs supervision practices
- Models of supervision
- Supervision tools and techniques
- What works well/less well in current supervision practices?
- What needs to change?

These workshops reignited the passion for clinical supervision within the group and sparked discussion, reflection, debate and the sharing of ideas relating to it. It became evident that even defining what clinical supervision was, or indeed was not, was not as easy or obvious as it first seemed. There were a wide range of perspectives and variety of methods and approaches to clinical supervision across the different teams and professions within Therapy Services. Having an external facilitator for these discussions was beneficial for the group as they acted as an impartial 'critical friend' questioning current practices and helping to find common ground. Discussions showed there were areas with good practice and areas needing more work. For example, some teams reported the use of supervision contracts, prioritising supervision sessions and ensuring clinical supervision was kept separate from managerial supervision. Other teams reported frequently cancelled sessions and being unclear as to whether what they believed to be clinical supervision was actually taking place.

A common theme which emerged during discussions was the confusion between what was considered to be clinical supervision. The distinction between line management, caseload discussions and planning, ad-hoc clinical or professional support, mentoring and supervision were reported as being somewhat blurred. It was clear some supervision sessions being carried out were management supervision sessions, or day to day caseload discussions. Whilst important activities to carry out, these would not in isolation meet the supervision requirements of the various professional bodies and the HCPC. The external facilitator supported the group by increasing their knowledge and skills regarding supervision, as well as challenging assumptions and current practices. This was valuable and allowed for the development of common understanding and agreement. This led to easier and more cooperative group working subsequently, when differences in opinion arose and consensus agreements were needed.

The staff who attended the workshops became members of a clinical supervision working group and it was agreed a project was needed to develop a therapy wide supervision resource pack with guidance, training, templates and tools. The objective of the group was to promote high quality clinical supervision and enhance the supervision experience which would in turn support staff wellbeing and ensure safe and high-quality clinical practice.

The Head of Therapies, having commissioned the facilitated supervision workshops was fully supportive of the working group, and agreed with the importance of developing guidance and resources. This support, as well as the expectations and accountability that came with it, was really important to ensure the group was given the time and priority it required, as well as the impetus, to complete the project. Additionally, developing an action plan and making a commitment to produce the resource pack with an external facilitator present, provided further motivation.

The process

The group's action plan had six distinct stages – reviewing current practices, exploring best practice and professional body guidance, developing standards and recommendations, collating paperwork and resources, disseminating the information about this across the department and then offering training to all staff in Therapies involved in clinical supervision.

Stage 1 Review current practices

Having achieved a consensus agreement as to what clinical supervision was, the group decided they needed to know what was happening at the time within the department. Were staff having regular, high-quality supervision, that they were satisfied with? A baseline measure of current supervision arrangements and staff satisfaction was established via a survey before making any changes.

The response rate for the survey was 31% showing relatively limited engagement with the topic from the therapy staff. Of the responses, 52% were from physiotherapists, 21% from occupational therapists, 16% from dietitians and 11% from speech and language therapists so broadly representative of the proportions of the different professions within the department. Interestingly 85% of respondents were band 6 and above, so generally more experienced or specialist clinicians. Without further investigation into this it is hard to draw definite conclusions, however, this could indicate supervision not being seen as a priority with less experienced clinicians.

The survey results showed that whilst most of the staff who responded (93%) reported they were satisfied or highly satisifed with the quality and location of their supervision, the majority of staff were receiving it less often than they would have liked. A high proportion (76%) had experienced cancellations of supervision sessions, very few people had clinical supervision contracts, or any formal training in supervision and almost all staff reported they would like more regular sessions, with more time to plan in advance. Unfortunately the responses were not broken down into professions or clinical areas so it was not possible to acertain whether one professional group was more satisfied than another with their current clinical supervision arrangements. Instead conclusions were made in general and applied across the department. It would be helpful if future reviews were able to be analysed more specifically in order to target training or resources more effectively.

Stage 2 Research best practice

After establishing what was happening in the present, the working group then researched best practice as defined within documents and guidance from the relevant professional bodies and regulators. Professional bodies included the RCSLT, the Royal College of Occupational Therapists (RCOT), the Chartered Society of Physiotherapists (CSP) and the British Dietetic Association (BDA). The relevant regulators were the Care Quality Commission (CQC), which is an independent regulator of health and adult social care in England, and the HCPC which regulates a number of health and care professions within the UK. In addition to the published guidance and evidence base, the group also discussed the topic within their own teams and professional groups and reported back about what was already working well for them, such as the use of templates for record keeping.

Stage 3 Developing guidance and minimum standards

Using the collected information from Stages 1 and 2, the group then developed a guidance document and agreed minimum standards for clinical supervision for use across all the professions within Therapy Services. This guidance document included:

- what clinical supervision is intended to be and what it is not
- types of supervision including the difference between managerial and clinical supervision
- models of supervision
- roles and responsibilities
- advice on frequency and duration
- standards for recording of clinical supervision

During this stage of the project, inevitable differences in opinion arose, such as whether it was the responsibility of the supervisor or supervisee to complete the paperwork as a record of the supervision session. Another significant difference in practice and opinion was in terms of frequency and duration of supervision sessions. In both these examples the professional body guidance either did not specify or varied with their recommendations. In cases of disagreement such as this, the working group had extensive discussion and in all cases were able to reach a consensus agreement or suitable compromise. In the case of who completes the paperwork, it was agreed this does not need to be dictated by the guidance but should be agreed upon and recorded in the contract of supervision at the start of the supervisory relationship. In terms of duration, a minimum of at least an hour was agreed, allowing flexibility if supervisees required longer sessions. In terms of frequency, general guidelines were agreed upon depending on a variety of factors such as experience, competence and confidence of the supervisee, alongside the complexity and demands of their role. The agreed approach was that frequency should be based on the needs of the supervisee, should be flexible (i.e. can increase or decrease in frequency in response to personal or professional factors) and should be specified in a supervision contract. The group agreed that whatever the frequency that was decided upon, the most important feature of clinical supervision is that it should happen regularly and consistently.

Members of the working group were keen to ensure that in developing standards and guidelines, they were not being too prescriptive and were not trying to develop a 'one size fits all' standardised approach. The aim was to clarify minimum standards, i.e., standards and paperwork that were consistent across teams and professions, so all staff knew what to expect and what they were entitled to receive. They wanted to allow flexibility within the guidelines to allow teams and clinicians to adapt them to the needs of their supervisees across such a diverse group of professions and clinical areas.

Stage 4 Collation of tools and paperwork

The group collected tools and paperwork from what already existed in the department which would help support clinical supervision sessions. These included:

- clinical supervision agreements/contracts
- session recording forms
- learning log templates

- feedback log templates
- models of learning, such as Gibb's model of reflection (1988)
- conversation starters/reflection tools, such as the Blob Tree (Wilson and Long, 2018)

This was all saved in a shared folder on the computer network and was easily accessible to all. For each record or document there were several template versions, collated from the many different documents which existed across the teams. People were encouraged to look through all the resources and chose the templates which worked best for them, adapting them to fit their needs whilst keeping the core content. Guidance for how to use all these resources was included in the planned training.

Stage 5 Disseminate across therapies

Representatives from the group presented the survey results, guidance document and resources at a therapies-wide in-service training (IST) session. This is a professional teaching and education session held quarterly with all staff from Therapy Services invited to attend. The attendance at these sessions is always very good with representation from all teams and professions, making it an efficient way to disseminate information across the department. Slides and information from the presentation were then shared department-wide following this session. This was a one-off information dissemination session, with teams encouraged to feedback to members who were not present.

Stage 6 Training

The working group created a short training package with a set of Power-Point slides based on the learning from the clinical supervision workshop sessions, the research they collected, and the guidance document and resource pack. The plan was to train representatives or champions from each clinical team within Therapies to then cascade the training to their own teams within team meetings or their own IST sessions. The slides included a reminder of the importance of clinical supervision and professional responsibilities and a review of the new guidance document and resources, as well as an overview of different models, tools and approaches to supervision.

Benefits to practice and staff

The working group successfully met their objectives – the guidance document and resource pack had been created and shared within the department at the therapies-wide IST session and via team leads, as described above. The cascade training package was produced and offered out widely, giving supervisors and supervisees an overview of supervision and the tools available to use. The resources were pooled on the shared computer drive for use in supervision sessions.

In general people were more enthusiastic about clinical supervision, several staff reported liking the more standardised approach. This was especially true for staff who rotated between teams – they knew what to expect, and what to ask for if their clinical supervision did not meet their expectations or the minimum requirements. Many staff reported realising what they had thought was clinical supervision was actually management supervision or more ad hoc professional support and were now empowered to address this distinction with their manager. Anecdotally there was reported to be an increase in clinical supervision sessions happening throughout the department, with teams and individual staff feeling like they had been given permission to prioritise it again. Staff described improved ability and opportunity to discuss and reflect on practice as well as address emotional wellbeing. Staff described more varied sessions happening with more group supervision, not just one-to-one discussion, and the increased use of tools, such as the Blob Tree (Wilson and Long, 2018).

Challenges and lessons learned

All perceived benefits and improvements were anecdotal, with a plan to carry out a formal audit of clinical supervision (now we had defined minimum standards) approximately a year after implementation of the project. Unfortunately, this would have been spring 2020 and the Covid-19 pandemic, and the pressure it placed on acute hospital services, prevented this from happening. In addition, by this point many staff in the original working party had changed roles, left the hospital Trust or were on maternity leave. Disappointingly, with momentum being lost and the immense service pressures, the old habits of deprioritising and cancelling supervision sessions returned.

It would be easy to blame the pandemic for the loss in momentum, however, I think this would not be the full story. In hindsight, the project and working group was seen more as a one-off initiative by both management and the working group, with deliverables and outcomes which were ticked-off, rather than a means to achieve sustainable culture change. It was definitely a great start – however, it lacked the long-term plan to help maintain it. Implementing a quality improvement framework, such as the use of Plan Do Study Act (PDSA) cycles (NHS England), would have been useful.

Even prior to the pandemic not all teams embraced or engaged with the new guidance and resources. The training was not mandatory, and some teams did not feel they needed it or were not interested in it. In practice, there were still blurred lines between managerial and clinical supervision, as well as what would be considered as general or everyday professional support. Some individuals were adamant they were getting 'loads' of clinical supervision but it was more just daily caseload discussions or ad hoc joint sessions which, whilst very much needed to maintain safe and effective clinical practice, was not strictly clinical supervision – a place to take practice uncertainties and to reflect deeply. In hindsight, I think supervision is such a fundamentally important thing to get right, the training should have been made mandatory for all registered staff. People who were not interested because they thought their clinical supervision practices were adequate, and those reporting satisfaction with their current supervision, would still have benefitted from a refresher. This may have opened up their awareness to any blind spots in their knowledge and skills – they 'don't know what they don't know'!

Additionally, poorer engagement from some teams may indicate their lack of involvement or consultation in the process. Although the working group was representative of all professional groups within Therapies it was not representative of all teams, job roles and clinical areas. In hindsight, the working group presented the new guidance and resources as a completed project, as the agreed way forward without considering further consultation. An extra step within the process involving wider consultation on the guidance, although would have taken longer, may have resulted in more engagement and buy in.

On discussion with team members there was variability with the amount of trust supervisees had in their supervisors, therefore, people reported not always feeling willing or able to be open and honest about practice concerns and vulnerability. This was possibly related to the skills of the supervisor to be able to create a safe space to facilitate discussions and reflections, as well as potentially the fact that many people had their manager as their clinical supervisor so did not feel safe opening up about issues which may affect their performance on appraisals etc. Specific training and support systems for clinical supervisors was needed to address this.

Working within a busy acute hospital NHS Trust there were on-going issues of time being too scarce and supervision still not being prioritised and cancelled when busy. This was already an issue pre-pandemic and was heightened in the extreme during the worst of the pressures. The Covid-19 pandemic also meant teams were working in completely new ways and having to adapt to rapid, unsettling changes. In the first wave clinical supervision was de-prioritised, along with all other meetings, at a time when arguably it was needed even more. Again, this situation heightened the already existing conflict within many healthcare organisations, i.e. the emphasis and prioritisation of face-to-face patient contact in order to support flow and discharge at the expense of staff support and professional development. Even if, in theory, an organisation fully supports the development of a positive culture of supervision, the demands placed on clinicians and their competing pressures often undermines this.

Further to the challenges described above, since the implementation of the Therapies supervision guidance the Trust merged with another acute hospital Trust – effectively doubling the size of the Therapies department and meaning a significant proportion of the staff are unaware of the documentation and resources available. This further increased the variability of supervision practices happening in the department and the complexity of creating a more unified approach.

The challenges encountered in this project are summarised in Figure 12.2.

Moving forward

Following the merger and appointment of a new Head of Therapies, I raised my concerns about the variability in frequency and quality of clinical supervision practices within the department. I championed improving clinical supervision to be specified within our department objectives and action planning, and this was welcomed and supported by all of the senior leadership team. Early in 2022 a new working group was set up with representatives from each profession and clinical area across the newly

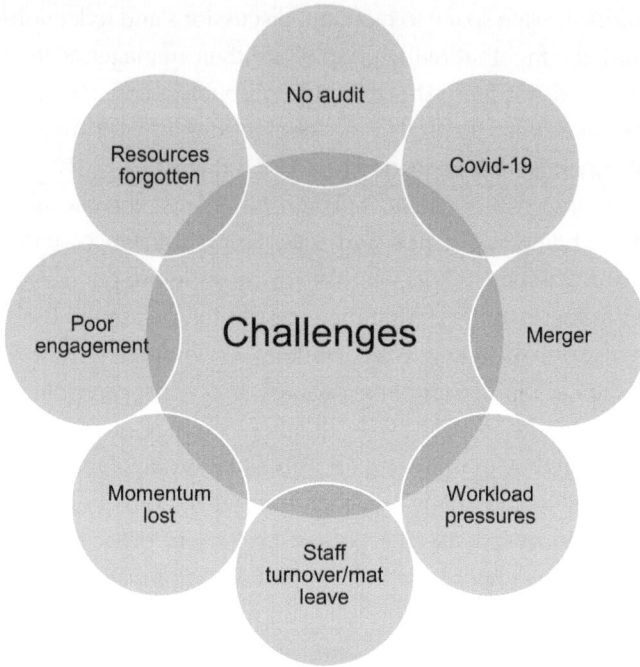

Figure 12.2 Challenges in supervision strategy development

merged Therapies department with the aim to re-launch the project and gain momentum again.

Although the group is aware that staff at one Trust has been through this process already and created guidance and resources, they were keen to not simply assume this was the best approach and there was a strong feeling it needed to be approached together as a merged organisation – taking the good practice from both previous organisations not biasing one over the other. The group were keen to avoid some of the challenges the previous group experienced – the most important being the sustainability of the project. The initial group was set up like a task and finish group, achieving their tasks and disbanding. The current group are keen that, although there will be very specific goals and key deliverables with task and finish projects, the Therapies Supervision Group should continue as a permanent group set up within the Therapies clinical governance structure. Hopefully this will ensure momentum continues with the implementation of any projects and that regular review, audits and updates happen, keeping up with best practice and organisational changes.

Covid-19 has shown how new ways of working are very possible and can be implemented at short notice. Supervision does not always have to be a traditional 1:1 session and we can be creative to meet the needs of the supervisee and the service. A key aim of the group is to update current resources to reflect this. The importance of having minimum standards and consistent paperwork is agreed, however the group are keen to ensure that there is a wide range of resources to allow teams to adapt flexibly to their own needs. Different teams, clinical areas and job roles require different approaches, and the aim is to standardise whilst encouraging flexibility – adapting resources to suit individual needs and avoid a 'one size fits all' mentality.

Ultimately the initial workshops and project, as well as the new Therapies Supervision Group are essential to us all as healthcare professionals. They highlight the need to keep the importance of clinical supervision at forefront of people's minds. To give permission for it to be prioritised and embedded into routine ways of working and our culture – to become 'just how it is round here'. Currently it still tends to be cancelled when service pressures increase and given the perpetual NHS pressures we are experiencing, there will always be too many patients to see. The importance of clinical supervision for staff wellbeing and safe clinical practice cannot be underestimated – now is the time it is needed the most.

Concluding thoughts

In this chapter I have shared my experiences and reflections on a project carried out by members of a multi-professional group aimed at enhancing clinical supervision across the therapy workforce in a large acute NHS hospital Trust. I explored what prompted the project and what stages were involved in implementing it. I then went on to describe the perceived benefits and challenges, as well as ways to move forward. To conclude, I share an overview of the key learning points from this project in Figure 12.3 and a detailed summary of these learning points in Table 12.1, for anyone who may be embarking on a similar project.

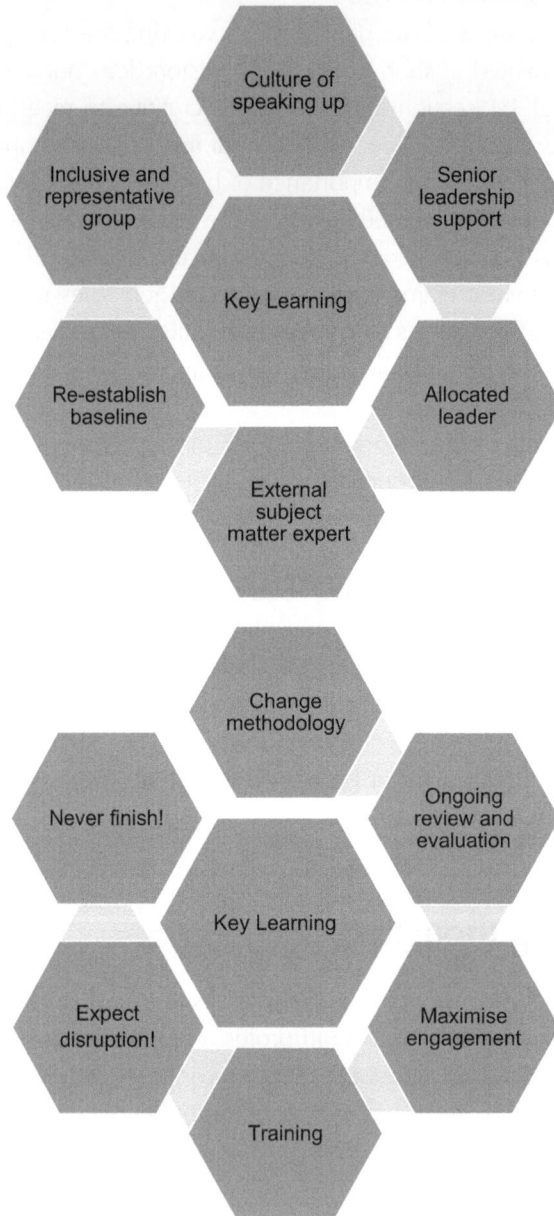

Figure 12.3 Key learning from supervision strategy development

Table 12.1 Supervision project key learning

Project Key Learning – the importance and value of:
Speaking-up and championing change when concerns arise regarding supervision practices
Senior management/leadership support and buy in
Having an allocated leader (or leadership team) to advocate the need for change, have accountability and maintain change momentum
Working with an external subject matter expert to support establishing common ground and provide initial project momentum and accountability
Establishing a baseline – what is currently happening, what is working well, what needs improving
Having an inclusive and representative working group, as well as creating opportunities for wider consultation
Recognising the difference between delivering tangible outputs through a task and finish group, such as the guidance document, and achieving momentum for lasting change with culture shift in order to embed in practice
Identifying mechanisms for ongoing review and evaluation, e.g. change methodology, PDSA cycles, audit, ongoing steering group
Maximising engagement e.g. make training mandatory, link back to HCPC standards and responsibilities, ongoing consultation and reviews
Training – not just to raise awareness of the guidance and expectations but to also equip supervisors and supervisees with the skills to make the most of their clinical supervision sessions
Expecting the unexpected! Disruptions, such as Covid-19 and extreme operating pressures, are commonplace in healthcare settings and must not get in the way of embedding and maintaining robust supervision practices which support care quality, patient safety and staff wellbeing
Not giving up and not expecting to be 'finished' – enhancing supervision practices is a continually evolving process and, as with all clinical practice, there is always more to learn and improve upon

References:

Gibbs, G. 1988. *Learning by Doing: A Guide to Teaching and Learning Methods.* Oxford: Oxford Brookes University.

HCPC, 2023. *Standards of Proficiency*. Available online at: www.hcpc-uk.org/standards/standards-of-proficiency/ [Accessed 12 December 2023].

NHS England. *Plan, Do, Study, Act (PDSA) Cycles and the Model for Improvement.* Available online at: www.england.nhs.uk/wp-content/uploads/2022/01/qsir-pdsa-cycles-model-for-improvement.pdf [Accessed 12 December 2023].

RCSLT, 2017. *Information on Supervision Document.* Available online at: www.rcslt.org/wp-content/uploads/media/docs/delivering-quality-services/infomation-on-supervision.pdf [Accessed 12 December 2023].

Wilson, P., and Long, I., 2018. *The Big Book of Blob Trees*, 2nd edn. London: Routledge.

13 Group Supervision
'A Woven Sculpture'
Ann Farquhar, Karen Cundy,
Sarah Stewart and Zein Pereira

Our supervision group has worked together for seven years. There are six of us in the group and in addition we have a group facilitator. We gather three to four times per year and meet for three hours. This chapter will describe how our group works and how it is different from the supervision we have accessed previously. The group has had a significant impact on our day-to-day work with our clients in clinical practice and on the wider decisions we have made around our career development.

Our group has members from across the UK and evolved from a shared interest in Personal Construct Psychology (PCP), an approach by Kelly (1955; 1991) that we are continually learning and experimenting with, both within and outside the group context. This chapter is not about PCP, and you do not need a knowledge of PCP to read it. However, for us the main principles of this approach which have influenced our group practice include:

- Credulous (active) listening
- Recognising there are always alternative ways of seeing and doing things
- Experimenting with new ideas
- Standing alongside someone/putting ourselves in other's shoes
- Viewing each person as the expert on their personal experience
- Using the key principles to relate to ourselves as well as clients and situations.

Of the six in the group, there are four of us writing this chapter and we are all speech and language therapists (SLT). The subtitle, 'A woven

DOI: 10.4324/9781003301141-13

sculpture', emerged from our initial discussions. It reflects the way we collaborate as a group and how this works organically to sculpt new meaning together. Throughout the chapter, we weave in the use of our own words via quotations (represented in boxes) and also narrative explanations.

> You get that opportunity in a group to learn about alternative ways of looking at something. How I can walk around something and look at it from different angles and understand it differently and I feel we make something from that as the group progresses. We make something together out of our insights, our observations, our reflections, the way we listen. And by the end we have woven something, sculpted something that we didn't know we were going to and so I feel like I leave with something really tangible.

Writing this chapter

Collectively, we decided to approach our writing in a way that simulated the organic nature of our group supervision sessions, using conversations and discussions about what the group means to us as a starting point. It was important to us to ensure that each person's voice was represented, as what the group means for each individual is different.

We were aware that, for some of us, the writing process would change the language, and therefore meaning, of what we each wanted to say. We agreed to video, and audio record our thoughts and discussions, and then transcribe the audio verbatim, forming our chapter around these 'sound bites'. This chapter is built up from these conversations, using direct quotes from our reflections to develop themes. We hope that in reading this chapter, you gain an insight into how our group supervision works but also how it feels, with the quotes from our reflections creating a sense of overhearing snippets from conversations.

Through these conversations, we identified some key questions to discuss in this chapter:

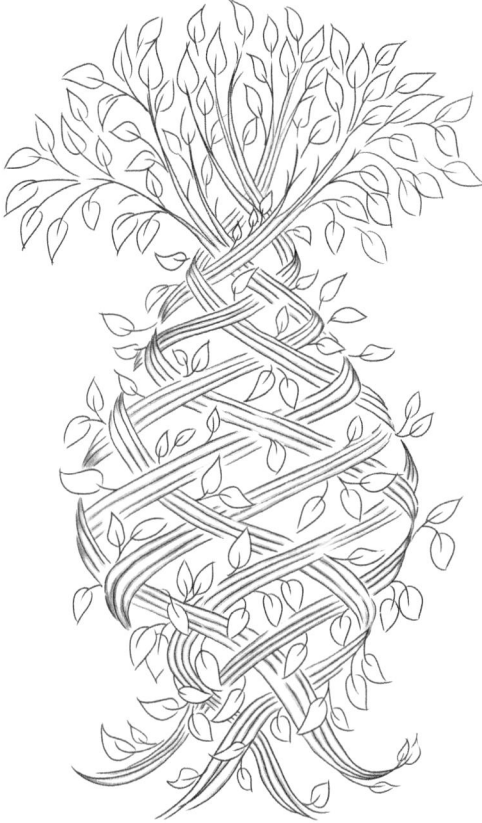

Illustration by Karen Cundy

1. Who are we?
2. How is this supervision group different to other supervision groups we have attended?
3. What makes the supervision group work?
4. What do we bring into the space?
5. What do we leave with?
6. How have we all benefitted from the supervision group?

At the end of the chapter, we have also identified some practical ideas related to the above questions. You may wish to consider, adopt, or adapt these points into your own group supervision context.

1. Who are we?

> We have total trust and as none of us actually work together which does give a different feeling, so we can be maybe freer in what we say.

We are a group of six professionals: a clinical neuropsychologist working in neurorehabilitation, a professional coach working in a corporate setting and four SLTs who all have different specialties and interests and work in very different environments, namely the independent sector, NHS (National Health Service) and University contexts. In addition to this supervision group, we all receive 1:1 supervision in our own clinical areas, which is a professional requirement. Those of us who provide one-to-one supervision for others, also access supervision of supervision. In practice, this supervision group works as an additional space to discuss wider issues that arise in our life experiences at work and beyond, rather than being exclusively clinically focussed. It does not take the place of other supervisory arrangements.

We did not all know each other before we formed the group but some of us had met previously on a PCP foundation course. Everyone was known to the course facilitator, and she invited us to form the group, offering to become the group facilitator, which we accepted. Our similar level of knowledge and understanding about PCP underpins our work together and has definitely sustained our group over time.

Our group members live and work across England and Wales. Before the 2020 Covid pandemic, we met in person at the group facilitator's base (for those who were local) and we used a video conferencing platform for group members who were further away. We consciously made sure we gave time and space for each member to take part. We continued to meet during the pandemic, and this was the point when we all transitioned to attending via the video conferencing platform. It was an easy transition as we all knew each other well. Interestingly, we reflected that once we had all moved online, this felt in some ways that we could all play more equal roles within the group.

The fact that we are not experts or familiar with the exact content presented by the group members means that we listen closely and perhaps differently, paying close attention to following an individual's line of thinking and asking 'genuine' questions. For example asking a question of which you do not know the answer and requires deeper thinking: 'Who has the power in this situation?' 'What alternative views might that person think about this situation?'

Our group encompasses diversity in gender, ethnicity, sexuality, geographical location, work roles and settings, and professional experiences. We have all come to appreciate the significant advantages arising from this diversity as we are exposed to different working practices, styles, and approaches which we can then all consider implementing in our own practice.

2. How is this supervision group different to other supervision groups we have attended?

> In my experience, in 1:1 supervision with someone more senior than me, they might ask a question they know the answer to because they want to test me.
>
> And actually, that's really key to what we do in the group – you only ask a question you don't know the answer to, it's about being genuine isn't it? Having a genuine interest, you only ask a question you genuinely want to know what that person is thinking about that question. It's not just veiled advice.

Through the evolving processes of the group, we have come to recognise that our supervision group is different from other supervision groups we attend or have previously attended in our separate work contexts. One key feature is that we all play an equal if different role which is in line with the concept of having more than one expert in the room, as we all bring our expertise of ourselves and our practice. In this group, the way that we listen to one another and consider a theme, a dilemma or an issue extends beyond reflection and reflective practice. In particular, we noticed that we are not trying to solve a clinical problem by asking questions that encourage linear problem solving. We value that the group does not focus on producing a specific outcome but instead we benefit from what evolves during the process of the group working together. We try to understand the person in context, then ask questions that enable the group member to step back from themselves and their habitual ways of processing an experience, to consider multiple, broader, and perhaps deeper perspectives within that context.

3. What makes the supervision group work?

What I value is the allowance of space, time, pausing, thinking, processing, working through, wondering, questioning and that only happens if you are given the space to breathe.

We don't want to muddy things by merging all our perspectives.

Firstly, defining the purpose of the group, the group values, and approaches that guided how we work, was a critical part of building a supervision group that felt safe and protected. We thought of a protected group space as one where we were supportively alongside one another and could reflectively explore dilemmas, themes or topics with openness and curiosity.

Each of us knew at least one other person in the supervision group and those connections helped to start the process of the group working. We have come to recognise that it is both values and approaches that make our experience of this supervision group different to other group supervision experiences. Early in the group's lifespan and as a continuing theme during the group sessions, we prioritised identifying the purpose of the group and this encompassed agreeing our group values and identifying approaches on which we would base our work together. The key PCP principles set out earlier was a central part of this and underpinned the process of each group session.

When we first met together, we had a verbal agreement where we all decided a number of ground rules including: the frequency and length of sessions, accessibility for all to attend, how to keep the agenda balanced in order to involve all group members, the importance of taking part and being fully engaged in active listening, supporting accountability and commitment to the group, and the value of having regular reviews around how we were working together. As part of this, we understood the importance of having a group facilitator and agreed that she would take the role of chair, organise the sessions and prior to the group session ask for contributions and areas for discussion to form a loose pre-planned agenda. We noticed that this approach ensured that no one person dominated the group session. Our group facilitator enables our discussions within the session and brings an element of teaching by sharing various theoretical models and techniques to experiment with.

This agreement was a very important starting point for the group to work well, so that we all understood what we were signing up to. As the group has continued, we have evolved how we work together within the group including a more fluid agenda, where each session builds on the last. For example, if something arises in a session the facilitator (or one of the group) might suggest this as a topic or theme for the subsequent session. We all enjoy the fact that there is an ongoing dialogue about how the group operates. Everyone has the opportunity to contribute during each session but with no pressure if an individual needs to be quieter for a particular reason.

One of the approaches we have taken on is that we are all explicit about how we view the group and the process within it. The group feels transparent and collaborative which is encouraged by the facilitator but adopted by all the members. We also agreed that suspending judgement needed to be demonstrated during group sessions, by others remaining silent and giving each person talking both time and space to reflect on their own personal meaning.

4. What do we bring into the space?

It's a Safe Space. I bring acceptance and an open mind.

What is brought is not always an issue or dilemma but a frame of mind which encompasses an openness to view things from different perspectives and non-judgemental listening. The values and approaches that we have agreed as a group allow us to feel safe enough to talk honestly about our work.

I bring me as a therapist, me as a person and know that it's safe to do so . . . that it's safe to talk about the feelings that my work evokes on different days with honesty and even when I'm not clear about what it is I am thinking and feeling but there is an honesty that I know I can bring and will be treated respectfully and listened to carefully.

Sometimes we bring ideas that can be vague or unformed but the way that we work through them together can clarify and progress our thought processes, in unpredictable or surprising ways.

> Each time I bring something different into the space and I suppose what I've noticed is whatever I arrive with or whatever situation or feeling or mood or scenario I arrive with I will always walk out of the space having moved forward in some sort of way and normally it's in quite a big way, it's more than I expect. I'm going to be totally honest, there are times when I think about attending our group and I think, 'oh my goodness, I haven't got the space for it, what am I going to take, I mean is it adding to my stress this week, you know, have I got capacity for it?' And I somehow always know that what it gives me is more capacity because there's always useful stuff being talked about.

We also bring an acknowledgement of uncertainty. We are all aware of feeling uncertain at times as it is difficult to predict what will happen in a group, how we might contribute, what we might gain. Trusting the safety of the group and the process has meant we are taken to unanticipated places which turn out to be personally relevant.

5. What do we leave with?

> Sometimes I'm inspired by someone in the group recounting their experience of trying something new out, I get some confidence up to experiment with an idea in a therapy session or supervision session and think, 'I'll have a go at that.'

What we take away with us and how it may impact on our work and lives is the most important part of this supervision process. There are many factors that combine during the session to affect what we take from the group, for example the experiences of others in the group resounding with our own experience, the power of suspending our own judgments during our listening and new questions being raised in our own minds during the group process. Through our conversations, we have identified tangible and less tangible elements. We identified that a key underlying theme for all the different elements we take from the group is the PCP idea of the 'person as scientist' and this involves experimentation.

For the less tangible elements, we may not leave with a concrete action plan, but something looser, such as thoughts and ideas to follow up or a feeling to shape into something we might try. Experimenting with an idea helps us to find meaning and see things differently. We then report back during the next group session. One group member explained that since experimentation is an expected part of the supervision group sessions, it becomes more natural to use this approach in work situations. This change in mindset then allowed more room for 'when things don't work out' and provided a resilience that supported their work in general and a feeling of being able to keep going in the profession during more difficult times.

> Professionally, I try out the strategies and activities that invite the family in, as it were, to say out loud what they are thinking, fearing, hoping. The group conversations give me permission to think about working relationships in new ways, think about how I want to work, what I bring to my work.
>
> I have found that the group has benefitted my practice in varying ways. For instance, the nature of the group has ensured I have had to routinely practice my credulous listening skills and I have then carried this forward when I am doing my own supervision sessions or, in fact, when I am having any interactions.

For the more tangible elements, experiments that emerge during a session for us to try when we are in our own practice, may include a specific technique or exploring a particular strategy in a session, such as more active listening, asking different styles of questions, suspending judgement in our own listening. These can then be tried with colleagues, clients and their family members or with supervisees.

For instance, in one session we explored using the Pictor technique (King, N. et al., 2013) which involves using arrow shaped post-it notes to map out roles or relationships. One group member described how they then used this technique in a session with a child to support a discussion about social communication. Based on the success of this, they used it with a supervisee to map out colleague relationships within their team.

Another example involved using a grid technique (Proctor, 2005) in the supervision group as a way of considering how others may have different perspectives. This was then tried within a different context with a client.

> Something I have explored in the group and used in my speech and language therapy practice, is a tool to support the client to think about how they see themselves from others' perspectives. With one client I have explored her view of herself in her communication group (in contrast to herself outside of the group). The tool is a simple table with a list of group members names across the top. I asked her to describe herself in three words in the speech and language therapy group, then in turn describe in three words, how X (another group member) sees her in the group and then how Y sees her etc. By breaking this down, it was a helpful way to support her to see her important role in the group, how she supports others and how she notices how she is seen as confident by others. The process of the group then helps me to reflect on the value and extent of the tool.

Sometimes a particular model is explored within the group, allowing ideas to be translated into practice. For instance, the facilitator presented Frances' (2019) continuum of facilitator styles for coaching and counselling to explore more explicitly how our roles in supervision or therapy change depending on the client or during a session. As a group, we discussed the different styles in the continuum: the reflector, the processor, the partner, the advisor, and the expert and how it can be helpful to have these in mind during sessions to provide support in the most effective and meaningful way. One group member reviewed how her supervision style with a particular supervisee tended to be more advisory in nature and we discussed why this might be. In the next session, this group member provided feedback on how she had presented this model to her supervisee and explicitly used it to reflect on their supervision relationship together.

Another model we explored in the group was 'The Wheel of Change' (Prochaska & Diclemente, 1986). One member then gave feedback on how this had impacted on their clinical practice.

The session we looked at the Wheel of change – it completely altered how I reflect on the complexity of change and therefore how I discuss a clinical plan. Change can be difficult. Thinking about this together in the group led to change in my sessions. I could slow things down to allow the client time to contemplate and I understood more and included much more of their perspective. The wheel also offered me a way of being more compassionate towards myself in terms of sustaining change. It offered a hopeful way of reviewing action and more importantly, inaction.

Experimentation may also evolve beyond techniques to affect our work more broadly and deeply, in a relational way. An example of this is using more creative approaches in our practice. We all take care however to make sure that if we are taking on a new technique that we are inexperienced in the use of, we access one-to-one supervision to ensure we are working within our scope of practice.

When others have shared their experiences of trying something out that we have talked about in the group, it has inspired me to be more creative. One group member described using drawing and painting with a client and how unexpectedly valuable this had been for both themself and the client. I have since used drawing/painting many times in therapy sessions with young people, e.g. as a way for them to describe how they are feeling about themselves or about their interactions with different people in their lives and how they view themselves at different points in time or how they might consider alternative versions for themselves.

Attending the group sessions has given me confidence to experiment with creative resources, such as using photos or buttons, as a way for clients or supervisees to express their ideas relating to therapy goal setting e.g. where they are now, where they would like to be and the alternatives. I have found the clarity a photo or button has given to the process of setting targets has been both surprising and inspiring and can be something that has long lasting impact with a supervisee because it is very personal: their own button/photo makes their words tangible and real. The group has given me a forum to bring my work using creative resources, and to reflect and evaluate together with other people who are also interested in working this way.

What we take away from a group is not always an experiment. For example, feeling 'lighter' or 'reset' may be a change of mindset that affects or even sustains us in our work.

I've never not walked out feeling lighter, kind of freer, bit more inspired, bit more bouncy almost. Cos there's something about the sharing, there's something about the no judgement, there's something about sitting alongside, everyone being their own expert and that lives in our group as a sort of underlying principle, and you can feel it.

Actually, leaving on a high note . . . is the enjoyment of loosely exploring all those ideas with other people in this safe environment that gives you that feeling of happiness and peace and almost like a respite and a resetting. There are things to try and move forward with, new ideas to think about and new techniques to maybe try and think 'OK, I could maybe try that with myself or with a client'.

The group flushes out what we need to think about and learn . . . I feel like the space created gives a rare opportunity to reflect deeply about my core values that somehow I don't think about at some other times. I think that is possibly why it I leave the group feeling like my lens has widened. I'm already looking forward to our next time, together.

Although our experiments are typically related to something that has arisen in the session, it can also become a way of doing things, an attitude even. Experimentation can underpin the way that the group asks questions and trusts each person to explore and examine their ideas, supporting the process of decision making.

6. *How have we all benefitted from the supervision group?*

Throughout job changes, life changes and challenges it's been a constant, I didn't really realise this but as we've been writing the chapter, I've come to see how important it has been to me as it is not dependent on where I work, what role I have, what's happening in my family life. It has been there throughout.

When I have had difficult issues, trying to reconfigure who I am, changes in my feelings of my identity – I have been able to bring these to the supervision group. Everyone's input, questioning and listening is enriching and practically really useful. I know that I can bring any issues or thoughts to the supervision group with complete openness and that I will feel I have moved on afterwards.

Because of the group I have made some big decisions about what I want to be doing more of and less of at work. The group helps me to reflect differently, and because of the group I have a higher awareness of what I'm feeling about work, and me and work. Group supervision for me has played a big part in how I take care of myself. It feels like a safe place, and I know it has been part of how I manage some of the feelings of burnout that come up periodically for me.

Being open in the group, trusting the others makes me feel supported in general and I think this has made me a better clinician all round. I want to offer the same support and openness to other people.

Attending our supervision group has benefitted each of us in relation to how we feel about our work, and how we are supported to manage the pressures and demands of work and life. Accessing a supervision group outside of our different and changing work contexts has proved to be a constant and grounding influence. Our group values steer us through sometimes difficult times, helping to prevent burnout and adding an enriching quality to how we experience our work. The diversity in our group and the advantages of having six unique perspectives has been invaluable, inspiring experimentation, widening our collective lens, and positively impacting how we work with others.

Practical ideas to take forward.

Setting up your group:

- Consider joining or forming a group that would complement your current supervision arrangements in your work context. A group could be external to your work context.
- Consider professional diversity which can add a rich range of perspectives that crosses over professional boundaries and areas of specialism.
- Be clear regarding the commitment you expect from group members in terms of attendance and their role in the group.
- Having a facilitator is beneficial as they can enable the session in terms of process and timings, support the flow of the session and gather ideas for the next session. Rotating the facilitator role from within the group can also work well.
- Agree whether the group is face-to-face, online or a hybrid.

Starting your group:

- As a group, create an agreement including frequency, location, how to include everyone in the group in an equitable way and balance contributions, style of sessions and a routine review within each session and across sessions.
- Spend time defining not only the purpose of your group but also the atmosphere that you would like to create, identifying the values that will influence how you interact.
- Have a conversation about possible themes or areas you can all bring to the sessions e.g. clinical issues, work life balance, dilemmas. Even if you do not bring an issue or agenda item, you do bring your values and willingness to listen non-judgementally.
- Establish how you will provide feedback from session to session. For example, using the start of each session to reflect on points from the previous session.

During/within the group:

- At each session create an 'agenda' which can be used as a flexible structure to support the process. Allow space and time for group members to reflect, think aloud and work through ideas and questions. Consider how to balance the agenda with techniques, tools and a more open discussion space.

- Take care with questions. Ask open questions that you do not know the answer to and are not veiled advice.
- Consider how the issues, themes, and dilemmas raised by others are relevant for you.
- Practice suspending and holding back your own views and comments when listening as a way of more fully focussing your attention on the person talking.

After the group:

- Make time to reflect on what you might take from each group supervision session. For example, thinking about something differently, revisiting a technique, perhaps revealing a question to explore further or moving towards experimenting with something from a different perspective. It could be just a change in how you feel.
- Conversations may continue to reverberate long after the end of the session. You might find an issue or situation that reminds you of a conversation in the group, which can be helpful.

References

Frances, M. (2019) *Personal Construct Psychology for Coaching and Consulting: A Continuum of Coaching Styles for Coaching/Consulting*. ICP International Lab Institute of Constructive Psychology, Padua, Italy. Coventry Constructivist Centre, UK.

Kelly, G. (1955/1991) *The Psychology of Personal Constructs* (Vol. 1, *Theory and Personality*; Vol. 2, *Clinical Diagnosis and Psychotherapy*). New York: Norton. Reprinted: London: Routledge.

King, N., Bravington, A., Brooks, J., Hardy, B., Melvin, J., and Wilde, D. (2013) The Pictor technique: a method for exploring the experiences of collaborative working. *Qualitative Health Research* 23, 1138–1152.

Prochaska, J. O. and DiClemente, C. C. (1986). Toward a comprehensive model of change. In *Treating Addictive Behaviors* (pp. 3–27). Boston, MA: Springer.

Proctor, H. G. (2005) Techniques of Personal Construct Family Therapy. In Winter, D. and Viney, L. *Personal Construct Psychology: Advances in Theory, Practice and Research*. London: Wiley.

14 The Value of Supervision
What Do our Clients Say About It?

Iain Wilkie

In 2017 I transitioned from being a senior partner in a large multinational professional services firm to becoming a self-employed coach and mentor. I was excited to build my practice supporting disabled people struggling for their voices to be heard at work, including those who stammer as I do myself. Early in 2019, I founded 50 Million Voices[1], a UK charity with an international focus working to transform the world of employment for people who stammer.

I was introduced to the benefits of supervision during my executive coaching training at Hult Ashridge Business School[2]. I quickly experienced how valuable it is to have a confidential, supportive and flexible space in which to discuss issues and challenges arising in my coaching and mentoring work. Consequently, from the start of my coaching career, I invested in regular 1-to-1 supervision sessions. Later, once I had built up enough coaching hours and experience, part of my application for accreditation with the Association for Coaching[3] required the formal review, helpful challenge and eventual approval of my supervisor.

I soon found that my supervision sessions were enjoyable too, being focussed on my clients' coaching needs and my own development needs. These were more nourishing conversations than I had experienced during much of my business career, where progress meetings were typically focussed on activity measurement and stretching targets. Starting out as new coach, the supervision I received helped me to become more confident in my new career, better at setting realistic working-time boundaries and more aware of my potential blind spots. These were all crucial areas to master as I worked towards becoming a successful practitioner.

DOI: 10.4324/9781003301141-14

Mentoring programme design

My practice has since developed to include co-creating and co-leading group mentoring programmes for disabled executives and for people who stammer from age 18 upwards. These involve between 6 and 30 mentoring pairs. The mentees are at a stage of their careers where they are experiencing disability-related challenges and also sensing disability-related opportunities, for example navigating the risks and rewards of being more open at work about their lived experience, building a better working relationship with an ableist line manager, or focussing more on the strengths rather than the limitations their condition may bring. These issues typically result from ableist working cultures in which the burden of navigating them falls firmly on the mentees themselves.

A key first design principle of these programmes is that the mentors also have lived experience including, for example, being the parent of a dyslexic child or the partner of someone with a long-term energy limiting chronic illness. For the stammering programmes, all the mentors stammer themselves and are aligned with key principles, such as living openly with their stammering.

A second key design feature is that the programmes include 1-to-1 supervision for all the mentors. Each programme includes a separate introductory workshop for the mentors and mentees. These introduce the concept of mentor supervision, its purpose and potential benefits for mentors and, importantly, also mentees. In addition to supporting mentor knowledge, skills development and safeguarding practice, a particular benefit of providing regular mentor supervision in such programmes has been for the mentors to gain the confidence to explore different ways of helping their mentees unlock particularly challenging issues and opportunities.

Burning question: Does mentor supervision benefit the mentees?

While the benefits of supervision for the mentors seemed relatively clear to me from the beginning, I soon became interested in whether or not it was helping the mentees as well. After all, the main purpose of the mentoring programmes is to support them. To help answer this question, I sought written feedback from participants in a six-month UK programme for young adults who stammer which ran in 2021 and was supported by the charity Action for Stammering Children[4]. Six mentees and six mentors responded. The quotes which follow below are taken directly from the feedback received. I had co-designed this mentoring programme but played no part in the supervisory aspects. This was offered by a speech and language therapist with many years' experience of working with people who stammer and an established supervision practice.

Mentee perspectives on the value of the mentor supervision

The results suggested that, although it was the mentors who had received the supervision, mentees had also felt several benefits for themselves as well.

> "I think my trust in the programme was definitely greater knowing that my mentor would receive supervision."

> "Coming from a clinical background myself, I found it very helpful to have supervision within the programme. I know how helpful supervision can be for myself as a practitioner and the effect it can have on my clients (in this case, me!)."

Mentees reported feeling more confident that supervision by an experienced practitioner was underpinning the quality of the mentoring they received.

> "Having the supervision was almost like having a safety net. To know that there were people behind the scenes who were on hand to support [. . .] was a real positive.

The mentees considered that the programme was of high quality.

> "The quality of mentoring I received was of a high standard and the answers I got back from my mentor were of a high quality and something I could put into practical use."

This was partly attributed to the support from the supervisor, who was regarded by the mentees as bringing additional expertise:

"I viewed the programme as more professional and also liked the fact that my mentor experience wasn't solely reliant on one person."

"The supervision provided to the mentors ultimately made the programme higher quality."

Supervision was reported to deepen the learning within mentoring sessions, in one case practising presentation skills – a particularly challenging area for people who stammer.

"I think that, because of the supervision, I was able to go 'deeper' with my mentor and talk more about the thoughts and feelings I experienced during and after this presentation."

Mentor perspectives on the value of their supervision

Experienced mentors as well as first timers found the supervision very helpful. In particular, they valued that supervision gave them a safe space in which to ask questions, explore new ideas, and to experience the benefits of pausing for reflection. As the supervision sessions progressed, the mentors themselves became more confident in letting go of the reins and enabling their mentees to lead the agenda and style of their mentoring sessions.

"It was a concern at the start that I was doing things right, but being able to bounce ideas off a supervisor, talking through strategies and hearing possible ideas was comforting and made me feel more at ease with the process and my mentee."

The reflective and open nature of the supervision encouraged mentors to develop their skills by trying new ways of mentoring:

"I had always approached [mentoring] sessions with a structure and a plan – I felt that was my duty to be a prepared mentor, but it came out that open flowing sessions could be more effective. I felt uncomfortable with this but decided to try it and indeed that led to a good session."

> ". . . the ability to flinch test thoughts and approaches with [the supervisor] had a definite positive impact on the quality of the mentoring I was able to offer."

Taking the lead in directing their learning process in supervision did not come naturally to all mentors. One mentor fed back that they would have preferred structured, topic-led supervision sessions, and might also have preferred group supervision. This raises the importance of clear contracting at the beginning of supervision, regular reviews and flexibility in how supervision is offered.

Other mentors reported how their supervision supported them with practical advice for approaching potentially delicate conversations:

> "My mentee had a very different approach to his stammer than I had taken . . . I was not sure whether any support or personal experience I gave would be helpful to him . . . Supervision gave me useful advice on how to broach this gap which worked well when I applied it."

For some less-experienced mentors, access to supervision was a key reason in them applying to take part and in helping them build their mentoring skills and confidence:

> "The opportunity to learn from an experienced supervisor and to count on their support was a big factor in me feeling comfortable enough to put myself forward for a mentoring position. It was a key part of my experience, and I'm convinced it improved my ability to mentor effectively."

While one of the most experienced mentors reported:

> "Without supervision, I believe the experience for both mentor and mentee would have been nowhere as rich."

Concluding thoughts

In my opinion, the feedback from the mentoring programme provides clear evidence that the mentor supervision enhanced the learning, development and mentoring experiences for the mentors and, most importantly, for the mentees.

I am aware that the cost of supervision is often challenged on the grounds of insufficient financial or time budgets. However, I would argue the learning and development benefits can last a lifetime and such costs are likely to be outweighed by the long-term development gains that supervision facilitates. The mentee and mentor feedback cites many different ways in which the supervision benefited them, both directly and indirectly.

Looked at from a different angle, to be working with clients without appropriate supervision wastes a golden opportunity to enhance the quality of the development experience of both practitioner and client.

Finally, looking forward, I have observed that supervision has also helped to build a larger and stronger community of mentors for the future.

Notes

1 https://www.50millionvoices.org
2 https://www.hult.edu
3 https://www.associationforcoaching.com
4 https://actionforstammeringchildren.org

15 Supervision in Advanced Practice
Insights from a Speech and Language Therapist
Lucy Titheridge

Over the next few pages, I share my experiences of being a senior speech and language therapist (SLT), who trained as an advanced clinical practitioner (ACP) in the United Kingdom (UK) National Health Service (NHS) acute secondary care service. At the time of writing in 2023, UK ACPs whose primary background is nursing, outnumber all allied health professional (AHP) ACPs such as paramedics and physiotherapists, or professions such as pharmacists. ACPs whose background is speech and language therapy remain in the minority (Royal College of Speech and Language Therapists, 2019). I share my insights about the transition into an ACP role and of supervision during that time. Some of the things I describe as supervision may feel unfamiliar. I include them because they are representative of supervision in advanced practice and because I hope my insights will be valuable for SLT colleagues as more of us consider career progression into less familiar advanced practice roles.

Advanced practice

In the late 1980s, nurse practitioner and nurse specialist roles were introduced to the UK (Leary and MacLaine, 2019). The role was not consistently well-received (Sitwell, 1988). However, these roles, paved the way for the growth of advanced clinical practice. In 2008, the Royal College of Nursing published an initial competency framework, which guided the development of further advanced practice frameworks (Department of Health, 2010; Health Education England, 2017). By 2023, advanced practice is recognised multi-professionally and across the UK NHS (Stewart-Lord et al.

DOI: 10.4324/9781003301141-15

2020, Fothergill et al. 2022). In England, the NHS Centre for Advancing Practice describes advanced practice as a level of practice while ACP refers to a specific role.

AHPs as ACPs

In England, a multi-professional framework (Health Education England, 2017) provides specific clinical, leadership, education and research pillar capabilities necessary for advanced clinical practice. This opened up the possibility of AHPs becoming part of the advanced practice workforce. The Royal College of Speech and Language Therapists (RSCLT) support advanced practice and consultant frameworks, recognising these positions offer innovative prospects for career progression and will contribute to improving service quality and access to timely treatment for patients (Royal College of Speech and Language Therapists, 2019). ACPs with a speech and language therapy background have increased however the total numbers are minimal in comparison to other professionals. SLTs in advanced roles often remain largely within profession and associated areas of clinical expertise. There are however a small but growing number who, like me, are in multi-professional ACP roles working in clinical areas such as frailty, stroke and general medicine, in rotas alongside ACPs from a variety of registrations and professional backgrounds, such as nursing, pharmacy and other AHPs. These roles integrate research, leadership, clinical practice and education development with the professional's area of specialism. In some specialisms the clinical pillar development requires becoming an independent prescriber, perhaps one reason why the number of SLTs in these roles remains limited as current professional registration for SLTs in the UK does not include non-medical prescribing.

The journey from SLT to ACP

In 2017, after 13 years working as a SLT on acute wards, stroke units and ear nose and throat services, I began ACP training at my local teaching hospital, working across the general medical wards and eventually specialising in geriatrics. A question I am often asked is why I made this move from SLT to ACP. To me this was an opportunity to learn new skills, maintain my speech and language therapy background but to develop clinically in my local hospital.

I was the only SLT trainee ACP at the time. Becoming an ACP combines master's level education, usually though completion of an advanced practice university programme with workplace development overseen and supervised by a work-place supervisor, which is the route I have completed. In multi-professional groups of trainee ACPs, everyone will have different existing competence and capabilities, some already at advanced level and others needing more devel-opment. For example, if the role requires advanced capabilities in wound care, paramedic or nursing colleagues are likely to be more familiar with aspects of those capabilities compared with an occupational therapist or speech and lan-guage therapist training alongside them. As a trainee ACP from a speech and language therapy background, advancing my clinical pillar involved develop-ing previously unfamiliar competences, such as cannulation, advanced life support and taking and interpreting blood results, alongside some which felt more familiar, such as cognitive and capacity assessments, supporting best interest decisions and family discussions, including breaking bad news. With different professional registrations and starting points, each learning journey will differ, as will the supervision that is necessary for any given aspect of capability; something workplace ACP supervisors need to be aware of.

The professional transition to advanced practice

The process of transition to a non-traditional role can be a huge step. Often a practitioner has worked in the same area for many years, specialising with a niche set of skills, as I had. Developing into an ACP role is recognised as both exciting and daunting (Moran & Nairn, 2017). In my experience, fac-tors which influence this transition include the diversity of professionals, the practitioner's existing clinical specialism and the infancy of the role.

Despite following the same curriculum and academic teaching, each ACP will experience individual professional challenges. These challenges may influence a successful transition into the role as a trainee and in turn as an ACP. Moran and Nairn (2017) recognised that many ACPs misjudge these challenges which can include testing political situations through to profes-sional jealousy or professional preconceptions which can be experienced as hostility and can lead to feeling isolated. I recognise these transition phenom-ena. As the only SLT in the ACP team I often felt a lack of professional belong-ing and ambiguity about my professional identity. While all ACPs in the team are doing the same job, each team member has their own view or ways of doing tasks due to their original professional training and skillset. It can be difficult to judge how you are doing if you are the only trainee from your profession with a lack of peers who share your registration and prior knowledge.

Of course, progression in any career involves moments of role transition, from student to newly qualified, becoming a team leader and so on. These transitions involve adjustment in role, behaviours, emotions and relationships with others. I like how MacLellan, Levett-Jones and Higgins (2015, p. 390) have described this as 'a journey from a place of comfort towards a place of unknown territory'. As SLTs we work with people who are critically ill and with life-limiting medical conditions. However, we are responsible for aspects of wellness, like the safety of someone's swallow or supporting communication so that someone can actively contribute to decision-making. As a SLT I might have been at a bedside as a person became acutely unwell but would have called for assistance and stepped aside as others stepped in. In contrast, as an ACP I am part of the clinical team who apply clinical knowledge and skills to stabilise acutely unwell patients and inevitably that also means being there when the team decide they cannot do any more for the patient. As my advanced practice journey began this felt like very unknown territory. Not only is the territory unknown but the skills I was acquiring and applying also felt much less familiar. The journey to advanced practice is sometimes described in terms of the progression from competence to capability where competence is about working to defined standards in stable environments with familiar problems and capability involves working flexibility and creativity in situations which may be complex and require, being competent and beyond (Skills for Health, 2020, p. 9). A trainee ACP might feel very competent at cannulation and have successfully cited an intravenous line on clinically stable patients but feel much less capable doing the same with a rapidly deteriorating patient and a team of onlooking colleagues. All health professionals recognise this sort of uncertainty but if there are few peers who share your registration, this can amplify your uncertainty and calls for thoughtful, compassionate supervision.

Making sense of the transition to advanced practice

The university aspect of development provides opportunities to look for theories and frameworks to make sense of the development and transition to advanced level. There are concepts in transition models developed in nursing which I have found familiar, applicable and helpful. It also shows that now I have transitioned into this role, I see myself very much exploring the literature of other professionals and not just speech and language therapy and how this can offer transferrable learning and contribute to professional development. For example, Kramer (1975) identified four phases of transition and this is something that is very recognisable in my transition from SLT to ACP:

- Honeymoon: excited, motivated
- Shock: vulnerable, more difficult than anticipated
- Recovery: clearer understanding of role and responsibilities,
- Resolution: meeting expectations, feeling more secure.

I recognise my honeymoon excitement as I embarked on my training. Learning new skills, such as physiological systems, examination and clinical skills, such as cannula insertion and taking arterial blood gases motivated me and gave me huge satisfaction.

I also have a strong association with the shock stage. These feelings lasted longer than I expected when I started my training. After that initial 'honeymoon phase' of excitement and anticipation, I experienced an overwhelming sense of fear and trepidation about the professional journey I was embarking on. Professionally, I had regular supervision and peer support, but often could not help feeling self-critical of everything I was doing. I reflect that being the only SLT in a group of trainees may have amplified these feelings and my concerns that all the nurses and paramedics knew what they were doing whereas I did not. Fox (1957) highlighted that uncertainty is an inevitable part of being a health professional so it is perhaps unsurprising that there are times when feel that I have not fully left the shock stage and it will take time to move on completely. My advice to SLTs as a trainee, would be to be honest and acknowledge these feelings and to take time to explore them in supervision with a supervisor you feel comfortable with. Supervisors can support the supervisee to recognise the inevitable ongoing uncertainty and perhaps professional anxiety, but balance this with acknowledging successes, existing capabilities and progress as the individual advances to ensure recovery and resolution.

Effective supervision can support the trainee ACP with these experiences. Supervision may not eliminate these feelings but can help the trainee to recognise that these are not unusual experiences.

Early in my advanced practice development, I recognised that supervision was going to be indispensable as I addressed my own uncertainties, just as this had always been important in my speech and language therapy career. Clinical supervision has been described as a fundamental component in a supportive environment (Sharrock, Javen and McDonald, 2013). For me, as an ACP initially being able to reflect on new clinical practice and new ways of working was essential as a focus in supervision ensuring learning from practice and reflection to improve my competency (Kings Fund, 1995).

Supervision in advanced practice

As advanced practice has developed, there has been a greater focus on what supervision is required (Health Education England, 2020). Advanced practitioners are registered professionals and not substitutes for medical doctors, but advanced practice curricula often overlap with those of medical doctors in training. SLTs moving into advanced practice roles should be aware that supervisors are often medical colleagues and for some curricula the need for a medical supervisor is a requirement. As a result, supervision for trainee ACPs often resembles the approach to supervision adopted with medical trainees, particularly in the earlier days of ACP when I was training. While the medical trainee approach to supervision includes things I recognised as a SLT, such as protected time reflecting on practice encounters with the supervisor, it also involves supervisory activities which can seem very unfamiliar to health professionals outside of medicine.

Although medical supervisors are experienced and have undergone supervisor training provided by their medical royal college, the likelihood is many have only previously supervised other doctors in training. For a supervisor who has previously only supervised trainees from the same profession, there is a need to develop awareness of differences between regulations and standards for the professionals they are supervising. Understanding the ACP role, the supervisee's previous professional background, possible fears and expectations and the trainee ACP's relative strengths and learning needs, are vital for successful transition to advanced level practice and to avoid confusion over scope of practice. Furthermore, the unique set of existing knowledge and skills each trainee brings can get overlooked when the supervisor is from a different profession. There is therefore a risk that the things the trainee feels most confident about get overshadowed by the things the trainee feels less secure about. A growing awareness of these considerations has led to guidance to support the development of supervisors for advanced practice (Health Education England, 2020; NHS, 2023). This guidance recommends more than one supervisor: a 'coordinating education supervisor' who supports the trainee throughout the developmental journey and 'associate supervisors' who support advanced practice development in relation to specified aspects of the curriculum across the four pillars of practice; clinical, research, leadership and education. SLTs moving into ACP roles will find such guidance valuable and that it supports discussions and agreements about supervision arrangements.

When I started my ACP training, a medical supervision model (COPMed, 2022) was adopted so I had a 'Clinical' Supervisor for each practice placement and an 'Educational' supervisor who supported the training pathway into qualification. I was not sure what to expect from supervision even though I have always had positive supervision experiences as a SLT. Supervision had been something I looked forward to because I knew this would be an opportunity for protected time to discuss cases, professional development, develop skills, learn and consider the impact of practice for me. Over my career, this had always been relaxed and with supervisors from a variety of speech and language therapy backgrounds. Having always had what I viewed to be good supervision of my clinical practice, including both one-to-one and group supervision, I was less sure about what to expect from ACP supervision. Would it be the same? Would clinical or educational topics be the only focus of supervision? Having been fortunate to have access to both educational and clinical supervisors, I have realised that I have benefited from both to build my knowledge and skills and to enable me to build my personal and professional confidence.

Reflections on medical supervision in the UK

In the UK, medical colleagues have developed ways of supervising trainees to help clinical decision making, knowledge and practical skills acquisition which are designed to help development but also to build practitioner self-efficacy and ensure public safety (COPMed, 2022). This is accompanied by an increased focus on the well-being of doctors in training (Health Education England, 2019) Although supervision alone is not sufficient for patient care, quality and professional wellbeing (Tomlinson, 2015), it is regarded as an important component of the safe development of trainees. As a SLT there were elements of this more medical-focused supervision which initially I did not recognise as supervision.

On reflection, I can now see the benefits of some of these approaches to supervision. Having an educational focus to supervision, particularly in advanced roles is essential to enable skills to develop and to continue to feel professionally safe in unfamiliar clinical contexts. For our medical colleagues and for many developing in advanced practice roles, work-based assessments are objective, observational, face-to-face assessments that must be completed and evidenced to develop and progress. SLTs moving into advanced practice roles will find these activities described as supervision and that they are very familiar to our medical and other colleagues. For example, a DOPS involves being observed doing a procedure (direct observation of procedural skills). An example of a DOPS is performing a skill, such as safely taking bloods or inserting a catheter. Another example is being observed performing an examination or consultation, a mini clinical evaluation exercise (MINI CEX). This is when you examine a patient and devise a medical management plan with your supervisor observing you. Lastly, a CBD is a case base discussion, when you sit face-to-face with your supervisor discussing a case or condition alongside opportunities to reflect on your practice. All these supervised activities are used to enable a supervisor to evaluate the trainee's clinical knowledge and decision-making and the safety of the supervised practitioner's practice.

Initially comparing these to speech and language therapy supervision, I felt these were not supervision tools and I felt I was being tested. However, I now see huge benefit in these approaches. As a SLT I sometimes performed joint assessments and reflecting on these were of such benefit for me, however it was not often that we sat down after and followed a structured format like a Mini CEXs or CBD as medical colleagues or trainee ACPs do. My development in advanced practice has convinced me these supervision tools are invaluable in supporting the formative and normative parts of supervision (Proctor, 2001) where the focus is on knowledge, skills and practice standards. I encourage SLTs making the transition to advanced practice to remain open-minded about these less familiar approaches to supervision. Reflecting now, my speech and language therapy supervision experiences were more often focused on restorative aspects of supervision (Proctor, 2001), how I was feeling about practice or a case and management. Should I return to speech and language therapy practice these work-based assessments are a supervisory tool I would take with me to strengthen my and others' skills in combination with protected time thereafter, as an educational and supervision experience that can be documented and recorded for portfolio and continuing professional development.

In advanced practice and medicine there is often a requirement that a specified number of each supervisory activity and assessment is achieved to pass a year of training and to maintain competence. Initially this felt daunting, overwhelming and time consuming, but it is now completely integrated in my practice, and I recognise the benefits to me as a practitioner but also to the patients under my care. Work based assessments are seen as valuable facilitative interactions between trainee and trainer with a high authenticity and focus on patient care (Davies, 2005). I argue that this extends beyond training to include all supervisory interactions including those that are peer to peer. Personally, these unfamiliar supervisory experiences have all been of huge benefit for my skill development but also my confidence and well-being. Being observed when I was working as a SLT was a rarity unless I was doing a joint session or had a student with me. However now, having a senior medical colleague observe me with a patient is valuable, although I concede initially it filled me with the uttermost nerves. Being observed is something I have become comfortable with, now regard as part of routine practice for me and has had huge guiding and supervisory benefit.

Something which also felt unfamiliar was that simulation is also viewed as a supervision and learning experience, again involving a clinical scenario being presented to a supervisor. Medical simulation is an artificial representation of a real-life clinical scenario, for example taking a history for an acutely unwell patient. This involves being observed by others or often recorded and then receiving feedback on how well you performed either during or after the simulation. Over the past decade, simulation has become recognised as a valuable learning tool (Scalese, Obeso and Issenberg, 2007) that captures individual outcome-based assessments (Langsley, 1991). In speech and language therapy, this is not a style of learning and supervision that is regularly used, however my experiences as a trainee and now trained ACP prompt me to question if it is something that would be beneficial for all health professionals in undergraduate training and post qualification continuing professional development. Drawing on ideas initially introduced by Kolb (1984), simulation is described as experiential learning, which encompasses a student experiencing and reflecting on a situation, before evaluating the experience into an educational episode. Despite this initially being an unfamiliar supervision style for me, the personal gains I have taken from simulation sessions are vast. Simulation activities have helped me to meet aims such as ensuring safe practice, enabling me to develop knowledge and competence and enhance safety of care in complex clinical scenarios as well as encouraging analytical and reflective skills (Department of Health, 1993). My experiences with simulation learning and supervision prompt me to think that the use of simulation should be more widespread in workplace learning as part of all professions' development and supervision. These more structured approaches to supervision felt unfamiliar to me as a SLT. However, the ways in which these were combined with more familiar opportunities to reflect and share my professional development concerns with my supervisor were vital for my advanced practice development as I will now illustrate with an example of supervision from my early ACP training.

Valuable clinical supervision as a trainee ACP (tACP)

One of my early trainee ACP supervision experiences illustrates the value of supervision which combines Proctor's formative, normative and restorative dimensions. This scheduled supervision came at the end of a clinically challenging working day. The supervision began with my consultant asking: 'How are things then, Lucy? What a transition for you!' In the context of my challenging and distressing shift, I could not focus on any of my objectives, such as 'becoming competent at taking bloods' or 'to develop an understanding of normal blood ranges' and instead, I talked about how I was feeling as a human and a health care practitioner in this role and how upsetting I had found some of the clinical encounters I had that day. I shared that I felt inadequate accompanied by an overwhelming sense of transition shock (Duchscher, 2009) and how much I had to learn.

To my knowledge, my supervisor had never supervised anyone but doctors in training, however his empathetic approach sticks with me as one of the best supervision sessions I had ever had. Reflecting on why that is, I recognise the skilful way in which he created an environment where I was able to share my concerns with confidence. I found it helpful that he continued to share his own experiences as a junior doctor, sharing that he had also experienced sadness with certain situations and often overwhelming fear about his lack of knowledge. Importantly he acknowledged that on some days he still recognises there are things he does not know. He shared advice about dealing with such sadness and reassured me that there will always be times when we all go home feeling upset. He advised me to worry less about my objectives for now and to focus on adapting to my new role and the transition from SLT to ACP.

It felt a bit unexpected when the supervisor then asked if I wanted to learn more about upper gastro-intestinal bleeding and to look in detail at the clinical details of one of the patients I had seen that day. He explained that this might help me to go away feeling more confident, knowledgeable and prepared for future encounters with this common presentation which I would often encounter as a trainee ACP in acute care.

Going back to my more theoretical university learning I notice how effective it felt to use supervision to combine time for reflection with some structured learning about a clinical concern. In theoretical terms the supervisor had given me the opportunity to consider formative, normative and restorative dimensions of the clinical encounter (Proctor, 2001). This also demonstrates the value of 'Authentic Professional Learning' (Webster-Wright, 2010, p. 112) which happens when the uncertainty experienced in clinical situations prompts conscious awareness for the practitioner to 'think to make sense of situations' (Webster-Wright, 2010, p. 117).

Supervision for development

This early supervision encounter fits with a developmental model of supervision which has been explored over the years particularly when examining nursing practice. Hawkins and Shohet (1989) and Benner (1984) describe levels of development, from 'child/novice' to 'mature/adult'. At that stage in my training, I felt highly motivated but had not gained the knowledge, experience or skills in many clinical situations or therapeutic processes. I had theoretical knowledge and experiential knowledge as a SLT but limited clinical experience as a trainee ACP in critical clinical situations that called for prompt clinical decision making. While I might have felt a mature/adult in my speech and language therapy role, I now felt child/novice as a trainee ACP. Supervision has enabled me to apply new medical knowledge in practice but also to have senior medical colleagues investing and encouraging me to reflect has been critical. I think as SLTs we are reflective; however, I have been surprised at how the different approaches to supervision I have encountered as a trainee ACP have prompted me to become increasingly critically reflective now as an ACP. I think this is multifactorial and is because of the different clinicians I work with, the different clinical cases I see and the variety of the role as an ACP. I have doubted myself so often but at times even having complements and words of encouragement during the course of practice has felt like positive supervisory feedback in itself. Being able to reflect and identify what you do not know is daunting but having constructive supervision guiding me as to what to learn has been invaluable, supporting me to feel professionally safe in my developmental role and confident that the patients I am working with are safe too. As SLTs our knowledge is so in-depth about specific areas, whereas as an ACP I have had to develop breadth of knowledge at an advanced level.

A final point is to reflect on is the clinical and non-clinical benefit I have had through professional support from the wider ACP workforce including, nursing, pharmacy, paramedic, operating department practitioner and physiotherapy colleagues. This has also been a learning curve. My ACP colleagues and I often refer to this as informal peer supervision. I notice similarities but also differences in colleagues' approaches. Some physiotherapy colleagues adopt a relaxed format focused on the supervisee's agenda while some nurses use more structure involving setting goals and actions to be achieved and reviewed. I have found different benefits from learning and reflecting with peers in these different ways.

Concluding thoughts

ACP roles provide excellent development opportunities for a range of health professionals and offer opportunities for widening patient access to services. Historically it has been nurses who were offered such positions, but over time opportunities have arisen for AHP's including SLTs to be employed in these non-traditional healthcare roles. Transitioning from an experienced SLT to a trainee ACP has presented numerous challenges. SLTs contemplating this career step should ensure supervision arrangements are in place from the outset. The supervision approaches I have described in this chapter offer a range of possible support. An important aspect of supervision will be for the professional and emotional transition which professions moving into advanced practice very often experience.

However, as I have described, there will also be aspects of supervision focused on knowledge and skills development which may feel less familiar than those we are used to as SLTs.

Given the very small numbers of SLTs in advanced practice roles and specifically ACP roles, supervisors will generally be colleagues from other professions. Very often for ACP roles, the curriculum specifies that the supervisor is from medicine and the approach will be similar to that adopted with medical trainees.

I urge SLTs moving into advanced practice to keep an open mind about the different approaches to supervision they will encounter. Gaining support from supervisors from a range of professions has widened my perspectives about the professional learning potential that supervision offers and that this may entail a variety of supervisory interactions and activities. I reflect that as the numbers of SLTs in advanced practice grows, there would be additional benefits in connecting as a community and perhaps providing opportunities for peer support and supervision.

References

Benner, P. (1984). *From Expert to Novice*. Menlo Park, CA: Addison-Wesle,.

COPMed (2022) *The Gold Guide. A Reference Guide for Postgraduate Foundation and Specialty Training in the UK*, 9th edn. Available online at www.copmed.org.uk/images/docs/gold-guide-9th-edition/Gold-Guide-9th-Edition-August-2022.pdf [Last accessed 20.09.23].

Davies, H., 2005. Work based assessment. *British Medical Journal*, 331(7514), s88–s89.

Department of Health (1993). *Vision for the Future*. London.

Department of Health (2010). Advanced Level Nursing: A Position Statement (online). Available at: www.gov.uk/government/uploads/system/uploads/ attachment data/file/215935/dh_1 21738.pdf.

Duchscher, J. E. B. (2009). Transition shock: The initial stake of role adaptation for newly graduated Registered Nurses. *Journal of Advanced Nursing* 65(5), 1103–1113.

Fothergill, L. J., Al-Oraibi, A., Houdmont, J., Conway, J., Evans, C., Timmons, S., Pearce, R. and Blake, H. (2022) Nationwide evaluation of the advanced clinical practitioner role in England: A cross-sectional survey. *BMJ Open*, 12(1), e055475.

Fox, R. (1957) Training for uncertainty. In R. K. Merton, G. Reader and P. L. Kendall (eds), *The Student Physician*. Cambridge: Harvard University Press.

Hawkins, P. and Shohet, R. (1989). *Supervision in the Helping Professions*. Buckingham: Open University Press.

Health Education England (2017). *Multi-Professional Framework for Advanced Clinical Practice in England* (online). Available at: www.hee.nhs.uk/sites/default/files/documents/Multi-professional%20framework%20for%20advanced%20clinical%20practice%20in%20England.pdf.

Health Education England (2019) *Enhancing Supervision for Postgraduate Doctors in Training*. Available online at: https://www.hee.nhs.uk/sites/default/files/documents/Handbook_Update_Film.pdf [Last accessed 20.09.23].

Health Education England (2020) *Workplace Supervision for Advanced Clinical Practice*. Available online at: https://advanced-practice.hee.nhs.uk/workplace-supervision-for-advanced-clinical-practice-2/ [Last accessed 20.09.23].

King's Fund (1995). *Clinical Supervision; An Executive Summary*. London: Kings Fund.

Kolb, D. (1984). *Experiential Learning: Experience as the Source of Learning and Development*. London: Prentice Hall.

Kramer, M. (1975) Reality shock: Why nurses leave nursing. *American Journal of Nursing*, 75(5), 891.

Langsley, D. (1991). Medical competence and performance assessment. *Journal of the American Medical Association,* 266(7), 977.

Leary, A. and MacLaine (2019) The evolution of advanced nursing practice: past, present and future. *Nursing Times*, 115(10), 18–19.

MacLellan, L., Levett-Jones, T. and Higgins, I. (2015). Nurse practitioner role transition: A concept analysis. *Journal of the American Association of Nurse Practitioners*, 27(7), 389–397.

Moran, Gregory and Nairn, Stuart. (2017). How does role transition affect the experience of trainee Advanced Clinical Practitioners: Qualitative evidence synthesis. *Journal of Advanced Nursing*, 74. doi:10.1111/jan.13446

NHS (2023) Advanced Practice Supervisor Capabilities: Guiding Principles for Supervisor Learning and Development. Available online at: https://advanced-practice.hee.nhs.uk/our-work/supervision/advanced-practice-supervisor-capabilities/ [Last Accessed 22.02.24].

Proctor, B. (2001) Training for the supervision alliance: Attitude, skills and intention. In J. Cutcliffe, T. Butterworth and B. Proctor (eds), *Fundamental Themes in Clinical Supervision*. London: Routledge.

Royal College of Speech and Language Therapists (2019). Policy Position Statement – Advanced Practice and Consultant Practice (online). Available at: www.rcslt.org/-/media/docs/delivering-quality-services/acp-position-statement.docx?la=en&hash=6903FF39923ADE84D31CB7FF61A37B6ECD25A359 [Last accessed 6/10/2019].

Scalese, R., Obeso, V. and Issenberg, S. (2007). Simulation technology for skills training and competency assessment in medical education. *Journal of General Internal Medicine*, 23(S1), 46–49.

Sharrock, J., Javen, L. and McDonald, S., 2013. Clinical supervision for transition to advanced practice. *Perspectives in Psychiatric Care*, 49(2), 118–125.

Skills for Health (2020). Core Capabilities Framework for Advanced Clinical Practice (Nurses) Working in General Practice/Primary Care in England. Available online at: https://www.hee.nhs.uk/sites/default/files/documents/ACP%20Primary%20 Care%20Nurse%20Fwk%202020.pdf [Last Accessed 15.07.2024].

Sitwell, B. (1988). Patients attitudes to a highly developed extended role: The nurse practitioner. *Recent Advances in Nursing*, 21, 82–100.

Stewart-Lord, A., Beanlands, C., Khine, R., Shamah, S., Sinclair, N., Woods, S., Woznitza, N. and Baillie, L. (2020) The role and development of advanced clinical practice within allied health professions: A mixed method study. *Journal of Multidisciplinary Healthcare*, 13, 1705–1715.

Tomlinson, J. (2015). Using clinical supervision to improve the quality and safety of patient care: A response to Berwick and Francis. *BMC Medical Education*, 15(103).

Webster-Wright, A. (2010) *Authentic Professional Learning: Making a Difference Through Learning at Work*. London: Springer.

16 Building Competency and Professional Safety through Supervision

Insights from the Specialist Oncology Setting

Kate Ashforth and Justin Roe

Across the healthcare workforce, the supervisory relationship is a critical part of ensuring individuals and teams meet the needs of the healthcare organisation through the provision of safe, evidence-based care to patients. As we write in 2023 with approximately 1.4 million people working in the National Health Service (NHS), it is the largest employer in the United Kingdom (UK). In addition to those specialising in oncology in the NHS, many more clinicians work in the third/independent sector. With cancer affecting one in two people born in the UK since 1965, many of those clinicians will have personal experience of cancer, either directly or indirectly. However, promising data have shown that in England, for example, cancer survival rates have improved by almost 10% with three in every four people surviving the first year after being diagnosed (NHS England, 2023). Speech and language therapists (SLTs) have key roles in the care of people living with a diagnosis of cancer and are integrated into cancer multidisciplinary teams (MDT).

We work at an internationally recognised specialist cancer provider in the UK NHS. Our perspectives about supervision have developed throughout careers in which we have specialised as SLTs in oncology with a breadth of experiences which span acute, critical care, laryngology, community and palliative care settings. In this chapter, we share our experience and opinions on the particular contribution of supervision to the development, psychological safety and competence of the oncology SLT. While we are drawing on our oncology experiences, readers may identify synergies with other complex and long-term conditions.

DOI: 10.4324/9781003301141-16

SLTs have an essential role in the care of people diagnosed with cancer and in particular, those with head and neck cancer (HNC). SLTs have been more integral to this patient population since the 1980s with the advent of surgical voice restoration (SVR) for laryngectomy patients. Given the significant surgical interventions and organ preserving radiotherapy regimes that have developed, the importance of speech and language therapy interventions has been increasingly recognised before, during and after treatment. Acknowledgment of the speech and language therapy contribution and reputation has been further embedded through increasing research activity. SLTs also have a key role in supporting people with shared decision making and when acting as advocates, for example in the context of communication impairment and end of life care planning.

Communication and swallowing impairments are present in a range of tumour groups. These include neuro-oncology, lung, haemato-oncology and gastrointestinal cancers, either as a direct result of disease burden or the consequences of treatment. Recent studies have increased our knowledge of dysphagia resulting from tumours outside the aerodigestive tract (Kenny et al. 2022; Silva et al. 2023). As a result, growing numbers of SLTs are now establishing themselves within other cancer MDTs working with people across the life span. In recent years, there has also been an increasing recognition of the role of SLTs in palliative and end of life care (O'Reilly et al. 2015; Roe and Leslie 2010; Eckman and Roe 2005). A recent study has explored the benefits of dedicated palliative care education programmes as part of speech and language therapy and dietetic student education programmes (Miles et al. 2023). SLTs working in these contexts need supervision which provides both psychological safety and support for the development and maintenance of competencies in a rapidly developing advancing clinical specialty. While SLTs are established as core members of the HNC MDT, we hear from other SLTs working in oncology and outside of specialist centres or MDTs that they do not always have access to the same levels of influence, supervision and support that we consider are essential.

Supervision in the context of specialist cancer care

Working in oncology is both rewarding and challenging. With advances in treatment, and changing patient demographics, specifically in relation to human papilloma virus (HPV) related disease, which is of relevance in HNC, there have been improvements in life expectancy with many people being cured of their cancer. However, there are increasing reports of people living with persisting and late treatment effects (toxicity) impacting significantly on quality of life (Paleri et al. 2014). People are also living with uncertainty with fear of recurrence being a priority concern for those treated for their cancer (Rogers et al. 2010). Despite the increase in HPV-related disease and improved survival, recurrent disease rates remain high at 20 – 40% (Abogunrin et al. 2014; Mandapathil et al. 2014). It should also be noted that in many parts of the world, non-HPV related HNC continues to be a significant issue (Prabhash et al. 2020). With the introduction of new treatments, including immunotherapy, people continue to live their lives with cancers which are treatable but not curable. There are also those who will not benefit from these treatments and will undergo palliative systemic therapies or best supportive care. Understanding the complexities of cancer, its ever-increasing treatment options and side effects is essential for the oncology SLT and supervisor. In oncology, and particularly as SLTs, we develop long standing relationships with patients and their caregivers, especially those who have been treated with a laryngectomy, who might have been formerly managed on a radiotherapy pathway prior to surgery. SLTs and patients form therapeutic relationships over months and years. This will resonate with colleagues working with long term conditions such as multiple sclerosis and Parkinson's disease. Just as with other conditions, cancer rarely presents in isolation and both comorbidity and psychosocial factors can impact on rehabilitation planning along with treatment toxicities.

There has also been a significant shift in public messaging readily available through campaigns such as early screening for lung cancer and bowel cancer and with particular relevance to HNC, the implementation of human papilloma virus (HPV) vaccination for girls and boys. The growth of digital information sources and social media has provided a platform for people with lived experience of cancer to chart their experiences and share a personalised understanding of their cancer experiences. Charities and health institutions provide increasingly accessible information regarding novel treatments. There are frequent reports of rapid developments in treatment approaches and high-profile individuals sharing their own cancer treatment experience (Diamond, 1998; Greenhalgh and O'Riordan, 2018). With this increased level of openness and awareness, patients are often well-informed with high expectations from their MDT, treatment and rehabilitation. People with cancer are presenting at a younger age, with many successfully treated and keen to return to the workforce and this is particularly relevant to those with an HPV related HNC (Miller, 2020; Zecena Morales et al. 2023). This may contrast with other populations where SLTs are working with adults with acquired disorders where the patients are frequently, but not always, older and nearing retirement. Working with people diagnosed with HPV-related HNC is an example where SLTs work with a socially diverse and often well-informed group of patients. We have noticed that this can, on occasion, leave the SLT feeling that the patient knows more than the therapist. In oncology, as with many other specialities, the SLT also needs to have the resources to manage families and carers. This is particularly relevant for those working with paediatrics and teenage and young adults as in our experience, there is the potential for the emotional burden to be greater.

The skilful supervisor will provide a high level of compassionate leadership in the context of supervision while also ensuring the SLT has the knowledge and skills to manage expectations and signpost people to appropriate sources of information and support. Alongside supporting the SLT with the emotional and relational aspects of working with these patients and caregivers, there is a need to recognise the importance of developing clinical expertise and to value transferable skills. This is so the SLT can contextualise prior knowledge to address wider complexity beyond a cancer diagnosis. By way of illustration, we share this scenario:

A new member staff who had previously worked on a rotation in an acute general hospital setting expressed concern about evaluating outcomes in the oncology population, specifically neuro-oncology. They felt traditional outcome measures were not suitable for use in this clinical practice. Supervision identified that in contrast to their experience in the acute setting with acute neurological cases, working in the context of deteriorating disease aligned with their experience with progressive neurological diseases in the acute setting. Supervision explored transferable skills at an emotional and clinical level. In this situation, it was important to create the conditions for the individual to question aspects of practice which may be taken for granted in other settings.

A key aspect of this as supervisors and experienced SLTs is that we create a psychologically safe space and model that we too experience uncertainties and remain engaged in our own continuous learning cycles.

Competency in the context of supervision

In our experience, we concur with the position that supervision should be underpinned by key components including teaching, clarifying concepts, critical thinking and modelling professional behaviour (Dudding *et al.*, 2017). This should be delivered in the context of a continuum of teaching, advising, mentoring, coaching and counselling with decreasing levels of advice and guidance. Ensuring that there is a coaching and mentoring culture primarily supports personal development yet goes beyond service priorities. Our experience is that a person-centred supervisory approach ultimately underpins organisational objectives and benefits both patients and staff. At the Royal Marsden Hospital (RMH) we use a range of approaches illustrated in Figure 16.1.

We have also moved to embed the four pillars of advanced clinical practice (clinical, research, leadership and education) across the workforce from the newly qualified practitioner to consultant level to support career development and shape aspirations. These pillars have been adopted from those that align with advanced practice models (NHS, 2017) and previously the reserve of the more senior, experienced clinician. The clinical pillar can become a dominant area of focus for SLTs working in oncology, and more widely, for many of the reasons we have highlighted about working in a

The continuum of support

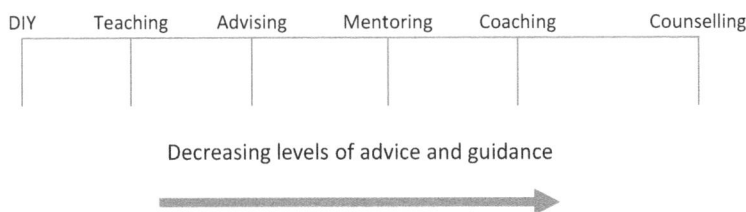

DIY	Teaching	Advising	Mentoring	Coaching	Counselling

Decreasing levels of advice and guidance

Figure 16.1 Continuum of support

Reproduced with permission of Steve Singer, Head of Learning and Development, The Royal Marsden NHS Foundation Trust focused clinical field where there is rapid advancement in clinical practice. This can be further amplified when the SLT works in a service with a specialist cancer care focus. With the four pillars forming the foundation of our supervision conversations, we can ensure that therapists are encouraged to develop skills and acquire evidence so that they are in a position to choose the direction that their career takes, recognising that this may not be exclusively clinical or limited to oncology.

A recent example of building evidence for the education and research pillars is demonstrated by one of our experienced (UK NHS Agenda for Change (AfC) band 7) practitioners who worked to support a less experienced colleague (UK NHS AfC band 5) to lead the authorship of an article for our professional magazine on a model of supervision for students (McCormack, 2021). Another illustration of the impact of the four pillars approach in supervision is that it has enabled two of our senior clinical practitioners to move from clinical to grant funded clinical-academic positions within our department.

The four pillars also provide a foundation on which to build skills and knowledge to balance the breadth of expertise required in the speech and language therapy career pathway. Developing competencies for the SLT working in oncology is supported by a number of profession-specific and multidisciplinary frameworks, standards and guidelines, such as Royal College of Speech and Language Therapists (RCSLT 2017) and British Association of Head and Neck Oncologists (Schache et al., 2021). While standards of care provide direction for practitioners to understand their role and expectations in practice (Schache et al., 2021), competency frameworks can be used to inform conversations around the knowledge, skills and performance required for them to be effective in their role as cancer practitioners. Through regular supervision, these frameworks support shared responsibility for professional development with measurable outcomes as the practitioner progresses. We have found the Macmillan Competency Framework (Macmillan Cancer Support, 2019) to be a useful tool to identify the level where the SLT is operating and to agree development needs based on professional skills, knowledge, behaviour, experience and qualifications. Including these considerations in supervision contributes to supporting practitioner well-being by building the SLT's self-efficacy in complex clinical environments. For example, in supervision discussions with our new NHS UK AfC band 6 SLT, we reviewed existing rehabilitation competencies using this framework to ensure they had an awareness of, and could deliver early, effective prehabilitation in the context of promoting enhanced recovery following cancer treatment. Using this framework to tailor our supervision ensures our team members meet competent, specialist and highly specialist levels of practice. The competence clusters include clinical practice, personalising the care pathway, supporting independence, interagency and partnership working and professional practice (Macmillan Cancer Support, 2019).

As we move from the overarching approach using the four pillars, tailoring to oncology with Macmillan competencies, there are core speech and language therapy skills that require development in order to work in oncology. These are specifically in relation to dysphagia and the use of instrumental swallowing evaluations including dysphagia, Flexible Endoscopic Evaluation of Swallowing (FEES) and videofluoroscopy (Wallace et al., 2020; RCSLT, 2013) and supervision is an important component in the safe acquisition and ongoing competency of these core skills. Figure 16.2 illustrates this relationship between the pillars of practice, speech and language therapy specific competencies and the Macmillan competencies.

We find that the use of competencies is valuable in creating professional and emotional safety in a potentially emotionally turbulent clinical environment such as oncology. In our view, providing space, time

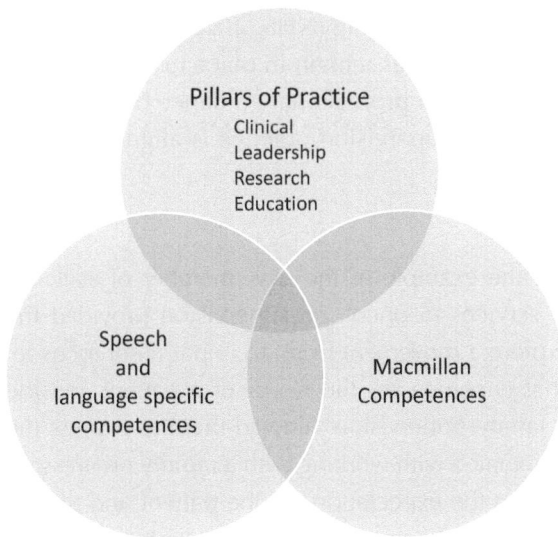

Figure 16.2 The interrelationship between pillars of practice, speech and language therapy specific competencies and Macmillan competencies

and encouragement for conversations about competency is an important dimension of speech and language therapy supervision in clinically complex environments where there is a rapidly evolving evidence base and innovation in skills and approaches. During our team awaydays, we revisit the concept of psychological safety so we can agree where we are as individuals and a team.

Delivering supervision in the oncology setting

In order to support effective practice that ensures safe, evidence-based service delivery, we use opportunities to deliver supervision in a group setting, individually, as part of line management, via peer support or interdisciplinary approaches. The use of the competency frameworks helps to maintain a clear focus on professional practice rather than more operational matters where the supervisor and line manager are potentially one and the same person. RCSLT supervision guidance separates professional and managerial supervision and we find our use of competency frameworks provides a way of differentiating these roles (RCSLT, 2017). This is particularly relevant with Health Education England (HEE part of NHS England since 2023) guidance recommending a transition from uni- to multi-professional team working (NHS, 2023). It is important that professional supervision structures remain in place to ensure individual clinical competency is met as per professional guidance but we also ensure that a broader theme of our supervision practice is alignment with the psychological safety principles.

Returning to the example of the new member of staff, transitioning from acute services to oncology, supervision provided them with a space to explore a movement from an impairment focus to a disability focus that encompasses the needs of a patient and their partner and young family. Supervision allowed them to express the complex emotions associated with working with a rapidly progressive diagnosis while managing the expectations of the patient and their family. The safe supervisory environment allowed for exploration of strategies to manage their own emotions and build psychological safety.

While supervision can be a tool to develop individuals, it also serves the need of teams and the organisation both locally and more widely. This ensures that well supported and empowered staff continue to grow personally while delivering on targets and organisation expectations. However, it should be remembered that it is the staff who provide the foundation to organisational success and particularly in the NHS where patients recognise that staff often go the extra mile (Brady et al., 2022). The Mid Staffordshire Hospitals scandal and subsequent Francis Report and more recently, the inquiry into maternity services in Shrewsbury have highlighted a breakdown of clinical governance structures and a lack of psychological safety with poor role modelling (Mid Staffordshire NHS Foundation Trust Public Inquiry, 2013; Independent Maternity Review, The Ockenden Report, 2022).

Psychological safety, the 'sense of being able to show and employ oneself without fear of negative consequences to self-image, status or career', is everyone's responsibility (Khan, 1990, p. 705). It is an essential consideration in all walks of life, but we employ this specifically in how we support our speech and language therapy oncology practitioners. Maintaining psychological safety involves respect, ability to challenge one another, trust, openness, a shared direction, good communication, learning from failure, and awareness of hubris. We create psychological safety within our supervision structures by setting the scene, defining the purpose and expectations, responding productively and expressing appreciation and destigmatising failure. We can continually evaluate team safety through staff retention, recruitment, exit interviews, patient outcomes, including compliments and our knowledgeable staff. We notice that the well supported SLT will be trialling new ways of working and encouraging constructive challenge. We have found that trusting the team reduces micromanagement and encourages growth. As team members become more experienced and senior, they may have less opportunities to get feedback than in their earlier career. We encourage shared responsibility for colleagues at all levels of practice to request and provide timely and specific feedback in the supervision relationship and ensure that this is embedded into the culture and structures of organisation.

A core part of our supervision approach is facilitated through compassionate leadership that encourages, supports and recognises a willingness to change. This perspective compliments our psychological safety approach. It facilitates a growth mindset method which is gaining popularity in health and beyond, for example in primary education (Dweck, 2017). Through compassionate leadership, our supervision approach has a focus on listening to, understanding, empathising with and supporting our team. Through supervision, we aim to make people feel valued, respected and cared for. In turn, they can release their potential and provide excellent care. Compassionate leadership results in a more engaged and motivated workforce with improved wellbeing and consequently, delivering high-quality care (West, 2021). Through formal and informal supervision and learning opportunities, shared solutions are sought to clinical problems. We use one-to-one supervision meetings but also other professional support opportunities such as joint working, reflecting on both positive and less positive aspects of clinical sessions. Using methods common to coaching practice, we invite feedback on our own supervisory practice from supervisees. Similarly, we invite feedback on our clinical work from staff of all grades in our team. This fosters psychological safety by demonstrating that even the most experienced practitioners are continuing to learn and evolve. We hold bi-monthly clinical case meetings to support a shared approach to rehabilitation planning. We also attend the MDT Allied Health Professions (AHP) neuro-oncology complex patient discussion. Our multi-professional AHP structure at RMH, whereby AHPs are in tumour groups as opposed to professional groups has really enabled supervision to become more organic and will be of greater benefit to patients and the SLTs themselves. We notice benefits in MDT joint sessions with AHP colleagues when our time together provides both a shadowing and learning opportunity for all present. The learning is strengthened because there is time to reflect on the session built into the supervision conversation thereafter.

'The expectation that we can be immersed in suffering and loss daily and not be touched by it is as unrealistic as expecting to be able to walk through water without getting wet' (Remen, 1996, p. 96). It is critical that the supervisor in the oncology setting recognises the potential for compassion fatigue in themselves and those they supervise. This requires an understanding of the signs and stages of compassion fatigue and to manage this phenomenon dynamically and that those leading less experienced colleagues also make and value time for their own supervision.

We also want to suggest that skills used to engage and motivate patients applied in supervision, provide an opportunity to employ similar and familiar approaches to support work-based growth. We model this in a way that is beneficial for the supervisee and is also transferrable to the therapist's clinical interactions. This includes motivational interviewing where supervisors can give feedback and guide staff to become more skilled (Marshall and Nielsen, 2020). This relies on core processes that fit well with the delivery of supervision and clinical development. For the supervisor it involves engaging, focusing, evoking and planning. Central to this approach is resisting the righting reflex (allow space to reflect rather than trying to respond with a solution to the issue), understanding and exploring the supervisee's motivation, listening with empathy and empowering them using optimism and hope. It is important to roll with resistance, share information and develop discrepancy. Along with the supportive nature of this approach, supervisors need to encourage a degree of challenge through feedback, accountability, agreeing courageous goals, introducing tension and moving from person-centred, to systems thinking and how their work relates to the wider goals of the organisation (Blakey and Day, 2012).

Workforce and career development opportunities

The development and retention of a highly skilled speech and language therapy workforce is an essential component to meet the ambitions of NHS Long Term Plan (NHS, 2019) with specific reference to cancer. Data tells us that there is a change in demographics with the more experienced SLTs coming to the end of their careers and there is a need to improve succession planning within oncology. As experienced SLTs working in oncology we recognise the need to ensure we have an inclusive workforce that mirrors and is representative of the community it serves and are engaged in developing community partnerships, for example in fostering interest in AHP professions and apprenticeships at employment fairs in local schools and colleges. These are contexts when we consider we are extending the role of the supervisor not just for professional development but to ensure the future of the profession.

There is recognition that the specialist cancer workforce requires strengthening. To retain staff in the specialism there needs to be a uniform transparent pathway for career development that can be supported within the supervisory conversation. This issue has been recognised more widely than the speech and language therapy profession and subsequently HEE have collaborated with clinicians, leaders (including the authors of this chapter) and other bodies including Macmillan to develop the Aspirant Cancer Career and Education Development (ACCEnD) (NHS, 2023). With the increase in cancer rates, training and education in this field needs to be broadened at all stages in the career pathway and foster wider, transdisciplinary learning. This programme will ensure that pre-registered AHPs and nurses will have knowledge and understanding about oncology and there will be a focus on those within the professions who are new to cancer. For those working in oncology there will be opportunities for enhanced training as well as leadership opportunities.

Macmillan, in conjunction with HEE, also devised the ProsPer programme, (prehabilitation, rehabilitation and personalised care for those living with cancer) (Macmillan Cancer Support 2021). This e-learning programme aims to support both AHPs and the wider workforce in providing personalised care and rehabilitation. It has a range of modules for differing levels of experience from the generalist in healthcare to the highly specialist oncology AHP. This tool will be of benefit to the oncology supervisor as it includes consequences of cancer and its treatments, cancer rehabilitation, management of symptoms and rehabilitation across the pathway.

Concluding thoughts

High quality supervision is essential to the delivery of speech and language therapy services. The process is a shared responsibility and SLTs need to ensure that they are offered and receive robust, regular and dynamic supervision to fulfil their potential and deliver a world class service to every patient.

Adopting a range of adaptive and flexible approaches and focus on supervision has never been more critical to ensure retention of highly experienced clinicians and leaders to provide a safe service. Robust supervision will motivate staff and address the loss of staff early in their careers due to a lack of compassionate leadership. Retention of leaders and supervisors is also essential and their supervisory development needs and opportunities for reflection must be facilitated. This in turn ensures their own psychological safety and pre-empts compassion fatigue. As models of service delivery evolve, including interdisciplinary leadership/ supervision, it is critical that a forum remains for SLTs to receive profession-specific support either internally or through specialist external supervision.

As we have highlighted, there are many more resources for the SLT working in oncology, both professional courses and those with a broader remit across the cancer pathway. A move towards a more resilient NHS has been recognised. While courses are offered, the SLT in oncology needs support at ground level in the form of their supervisor. With a focus on the critical question asked of our patients, 'what matters to you?', we have found that in our own practice, this question can also be asked of those we supervise (Barry and Edgman-Levitan, 2012).

References

Abogunrin, S., Di Tanna, G. L., Keeping, S. et al. (2014) Prevalence of human papillomavirus in head and neck cancers in European populations: a meta-analysis. *BMC Cancer*, 14, 968. https://doi.org/10.1186/1471-2407-14-968

Barry, M. J. and Edgman-Levitan, S. (2012) Shared decision making: The pinnacle patient centered care. *The New England Journal of Medicine*, 366(9), 780–781.

Blakey, J. and Day, I. (2012) *Challenging Coaching. Going Beyond Traditional Coaching to Face the FACTS*. London: Nicholas Brealey Publishing.

Brady, G. C., Ashforth, K., Cowan-Dickie, S., Dewhurst, S., Harris, N., Monteiro, A., Sandsund, C., and Roe, J. (2022). An evaluation of the provision of oncology rehabilitation services via telemedicine using a participatory design approach. *Support Care Cancer*, 30(2), 1655–1662. doi:10.1007/s00520-021-06552-8

Dweck, C. (2017) *Mindset: The New Psychology of Success*, 6th edn. New York: Random House

Diamond, J. C. (1998) *Because Cowards Get Cancer Too*. London: Vermillion.

Dudding, C. C., McCready, V., Nunez, L. M. and Procaccini, S. J. (2017) Clinical supervision in speech-language pathology and audiology in the United States: Development of a professional specialty. *The Clinical Supervisor*, 36(2),161–181. doi:10.1080/07325223.2017.1377663.

Eckman S. and Roe J. (2005) Speech and language therapists in palliative care: What do we have to offer? *Int J Palliat Nurs*, 11(4), 179–181. doi:10.12968/ijpn.11.4.28783.

Greenhalgh, T. and O'Riordan, L. (2018) *The Complete Guide to Breast Cancer*. London: Vermillion.

Kenny, C., Regan, J., Balding, L., Higgins, S., O'Leary, N., Kelleher, F., McDermott, R., Armstrong, J., Mihai, A., Tiernan, E., Westrup, J., Thirion, P., and Walsh, D. (2022) Dysphagia in solid tumors outside the head, neck or upper GI tract: Clinical characteristics. *J Pain Symptom Manage*, 64(6), 546–554. doi:10.1016/j.jpainsymman.2022.08.019.

Khan, W. A. (1990) Psychological conditions of personal engagement and disengagement at work. *Academy of Management Journal*, 33(4), 692–724.

Macmillan Cancer Support (2019) The Macmillan Allied Health Professions Competence Framework for those working with people affected by cancer.

Macmillan Cancer Support. Available online at: https://www.macmillan.org.uk/_images/allied-health-professions-framework_tcm9-314735.pdf [Last accessed 30 January 2024].

Macmillan Cancer Support (2021) ProsPer Programme (Prehabilitation, Rehabilitation and Personalised Care for those Living with Cancer. Available online at: www.e-lfh.org.uk/wp-content/uploads/2022/04/Macmillan_Toolkit_2021_V9 Reduced.pdf [Last accessed 04 January 2024].

Mandapathil, M., Roessler, M., Werner, J. A., Silver, C. E., Rinaldo, A., and Ferlito, A. (2014) Salvage surgery for head and neck squamous cell carcinoma. *Eur Arch Otorhinolaryngol*, 271(7), 1845–1850. doi:10.1007/s00405-014-3043-1.

Marshall, C. and Nielsen, A. S. (2020) *Motivational Interviewing for Leaders in the Helping Professions: Facilitating Change in Organizations.* Guilford Press.

McCormack, G. (2021) The pick n' mix practice educator p. 23–26. Bulletin of the Royal College of Speech and Language Therapists, Spring.

Mid Staffordshire NHS Foundation Trust Public Inquiry (2013). *Report of the Mid Staffordshire NHS Foundation Trust Public Inquiry: Executive summary* (HC 947). The Stationery Office. Available online at: https://assets.publishing.service.gov.uk/government/uploads/system/uploads/attachment_data/file/279124/0947.pdf

Miles, A., Brady, A., Friary, P., Sekula, J., Wallis, C., and Jackson, B. (2023) Implementing an interprofessional palliative care education program to speech-language therapy and dietetic students. *J Interprof Care*, 37(6), 964–973. doi:10.1080/13561820.2023.2203731.

Miller, A. (2020) Returning to work after head and neck cancer. *Curr Opin Otolaryngol Head Neck Surg*, 28(3), 155–160. doi:10.1097/MOO.0000000000000628.

NHS (2017) Multiprofessional framework for advanced clinical practice in England. Available online at: www.hee.nhs.uk/sites/default/files/documents/multi-professional-frameworkforadvancedclinicalpracticeinengland.pdf [Last accessed 04 June 2023].

NHS (2023) Aspirant Cancer Career and Education Development Programme (ACCEND) Available online at: www.hee.nhs.uk/our-work/cancer-diagnostics/aspirant-cancer-career-education-development-programme [Last accessed: 04 January 2024].

NHS (2019) The NHS Long Term Plan. Available online at: www.longtermplan.nhs.uk/wp-content/uploads/2019/08/nhs-long-term-plan-version-1.2.pdf [Last accessed 30 January 2024].

NHS England (2023) Cancer survival: index for sub-integrated care boards, 2005 to 2020. Available online at: https://digital.nhs.uk/data-and-information/publications/statistical/cancer-survival-in-england/index-for-sub-integrated-care-boards-2005-to-2020#top [Last accessed: 16 January 2024].

O'Reilly, A. C. and Walshe, M. (2015) Perspectives on the role of the speech and language therapist in palliative care: An international survey. *Palliat Med*, 29(8), 756–761. doi:10.1177/0269216315575678.

Independent Maternity Review (2022). Ockenden report – Final: Findings, conclusions, and essential actions from the independent review of maternity services at the Shrewsbury and Telford Hospital. NHS Trust (HC 1219). Crown.

Paleri, V., Roe, J. W., Strojan, P., Corry, J., Grégoire, V., Hamoir, M., Eisbruch, A., Mendenhall, W. M., Silver, C. E., Rinaldo, A., Takes, R. P. and Ferlito, A. (2014)

Strategies to reduce long-term postchemoradiation dysphagia in patients with head and neck cancer: an evidence-based review. *Head Neck*, 36(3), 431–443. doi:10.1002/hed.23251.

Prabhash, K., Babu, G. Chaturvedi, P., Kuriakose, M., Birur, P., Anand, A. K., Kaushal, A., Mahajan, A., Syiemlieh, J., Singhal, M., Gairola, M., Ramachandra, P., Goyal, S., John, S., Nayyar, R., Patil, V. M., Rao, V., Roshan, V. and Rath, G. K. (2020) Indian clinical practice consensus guidelines for the management of squamous cell carcinoma of head and neck. *Indian Journal of Cancer*, 57(Suppl 1), S1–S5. doi:10.4103/0019-509X.278971

Remen, R. N. (1996). *Kitchen Table Wisdom: Stories That Heal*. Riverhead Books.

Roe, J. W. and Leslie, P. (2010) Beginning of the end? Ending the therapeutic relationship in palliative care. *Int J Speech Lang Pathol*, 12(4), 304–088. doi:10.3109/17549507.2010.485330.

Rogers, S. N., Scott, B., Lowe, D., Ozakinci, G., and Humphris, G. M. (2010) Fear of recurrence following head and neck cancer in the outpatient clinic. *Eur Arch Otorhinolaryngol*, 267(12):1943–1949. doi:10.1007/s00405-010-1307-y.

Royal College of Speech and Language Therapists (RCSLT) (2013) Videofluoroscopic evaluation of oropharyngeal swallowing function (VFS): The role of speech and language therapists. RCSLT Position Paper 2013. London: RCSLT

Royal College of Speech and Language Therapists (RCSLT) (2017). Supervision for Speech and Language Therapists. Available online at: www.rcslt.org/wp-content/uploads/media/docs/delivering-quality-services/supervision-summary-for-speech-and-language-therapists.pdf

Schache, A., Kerawala, C., Ahmed, O., Brennan, P. A., Cook, F., Garrett, M., Homer, J., Hughes, C., Mayland, C., Mihai, R., Newbold, K., O'Hara, J., Roe, J., Sibtain, A., Smith, M., Thavaraj, S., Weller, A., Winter, L., Young, V. and Winter, S. C. (2021) British Association of Head and Neck Oncologists (BAHNO) standards. *J Oral Pathol Med*, 50(3):262–273. doi:10.1111/jop.13161.

Silva, D. N. M., Vicente, L. C. C., Glória, V. L. P. and de Lima Friche, A. A. (2023) Swallowing disorders and mortality in adults with advanced cancer outside the head and neck and upper gastrointestinal tract: a systematic review. *BMC Palliat Care*, 22(1), 150. doi:10.1186/s12904-023-01268-4.

Wallace, S., McLaughlin, C., Clayton, J., Coffey, M., Ellis, J., Haag, R., Howard, A., Marks, H. and Zorko, R. (2020) Fibreoptic Endoscopic evaluation of Swallowing (FEES): The role of speech and language therapy. London: Royal College of Speech and Language Therapists, Position paper.

West, M. A. (2021) *Compassionate Leadership: Sustaining Wisdom, Humanity and Presence in Health and Social Care*. Swirling Leaf Press.

Zecena Morales, C., Lisy, K., McDowell, L., Piper, A. and Jefford, M. (2023) Return to work in head and neck cancer survivors: A systematic review. *J Cancer Surviv*, 17(2), 468–483. doi:10.1007/s11764-022-01298-6.

17 Peer Group Supervision
Drawing on Collective Knowledge

Kate Balzer, Claire Farrington-Douglas and Mary Ganpatsingh

When considering arrangements for supervision, there might be a tendency to focus on one-to-one professional supervision, either because it fits with the organisation that you work for or is the way in which supervision is typically described. In the Royal College of Speech and Language Therapists (RCSLT) 2017 document 'Information on Supervision', one-to-one supervision is defined as one of several forms of professional supervision, along with peer, peer group and group supervision. The aim of professional supervision is to provide a safe and reflective space where the supervisee can discuss professional and ethical issues. The recommendation is that a speech and language therapist (SLT) will receive at least one hour of professional supervision every four to six weeks but the way in which this professional supervision is received can be tailored to the individual needs of the clinician. With this in mind and the possibility of 10–15 hours of supervision a year, peer group supervision might be accessed alongside one-to-one supervision.

In this chapter, we each share our history of professional supervision before describing why and how we formed a peer group supervision triad in 2020. We share what we have learnt about peer group supervision, how it differs from other forms of professional supervision and the unique aspects of supervision with a group of peers. We describe the ways in which our supervision and clinical skills have developed through our experience of peer group supervision. We detail how we contracted together and finish by sharing some considerations for setting up a peer supervision group with guidance about how you can access peer group supervision yourself.

DOI: 10.4324/9781003301141-17

Forming a peer supervision group

We will begin by sharing our personal supervision stories to explain how we came to form a peer supervision group.

Claire's story

Throughout my career as a SLT, I have been inspired by supervisors who supported me to think deeply about my clinical practice and my support needs as I work through the challenges of my work. I have reflected on my role within complex teams and developed my self-awareness. When I took on a leadership role, my supervision became more line-management focused so I sought out external supervision to ensure my clinical development needs were met.

I have been developing my skills as a supervisor with students, assistants and SLTs, as well as with social workers and psychotherapists. I have enjoyed developing my style of supervision. My ethos is to facilitate an authentic, open and reflective practice of supervision.

Earlier in my career I attended a counselling skills course for SLTs to develop my listening, facilitation and questioning skills, which proved valuable in my clinical and supervisory practice. More recently I have experimented with incorporating principles from personal construct psychology (Kelly, 1955/1991) into my practice. I have also attended supervision training days that involved practice and feedback, which is a particularly useful learning process. I now see every supervisory experience as an opportunity to hone my skills and, as a result, my supervision work is a highlight of my role. I have developed an ability to reflect and process simultaneously so that I can proactively work alongside someone as they navigate their issue or scenario.

Following an advanced supervision course, I decided to establish a peer supervision group to support ongoing development of my clinical practice and supervision skills. I was keen to find a space where I could experiment with different supervision tools and techniques and receive feedback on them whilst addressing clinical challenges from my work and those of the other group members. I reached out to Mary, who was also on the supervision training, as I knew she was interested in developing the same skills. I was open to a peer supervision group with people from other specialisms but chose to develop the group with two SLTs in the brain injury field like myself.

At our first meeting as a triad, I felt excited about setting up this peer relationship. Through our regular peer group supervision sessions and writing this chapter we have developed our supervisory relationship and reflected more deeply on the processes at play in supervision.

Mary's story

Early on in my career I received managerial supervision but had limited access to professional supervision. When I became the most senior SLT in a department, my organisation supported me to find an external supervisor so that I could further develop my clinical and leadership skills for the role. Receiving one-to-one professional supervision inspired me to invest more time and energy in understanding supervision practice because I experienced the benefit of the formative, normative and restorative aspects of supervision (Proctor, 1986).

Recently my supervisor and I re-contracted because we had been meeting together for over a decade and both our circumstances had changed. Although I was content and comfortable with the arrangement and did not want to lose connection with my supervisor, this process of re-contracting gave me an opportunity to review my supervisory needs. I became open to exploring new possibilities. One significant shift was the realisation that you can receive supervision in multiple ways, simultaneously.

I was already interested in exploring supervision in the context of a peer group. As an independent practitioner, I anticipated that it would be a good way to connect with therapists doing the same kind of work. I hoped a peer group would provide not only a supportive, reflective and challenging environment to discuss my clinical caseload, but also to explore how supervision works when there is more than one person meeting. In the past, I had benefitted from group supervision where a group of colleagues met to discuss some issues with an external supervisor, but had never received peer group supervision, where a group of peers rotate the role of supervisor and supervisee. Confident that I would be able to build on the existing supervision skills I had honed in the one-to-one context, I was keen to try peer group supervision. It was at this time that Claire invited me to consider forming a group, so I immediately took up the opportunity.

Already the experience has allowed me to refine my supervision skills and decide how I use my supervision time across two one-to-one arrangements and the peer group we write about here. With Kate and Claire, I have benefitted from talking about clinical issues with peers and find that our discussions bring about a broader and deeper understanding of any topic at hand.

Kate's story

I have worked in various settings within the UK National Health Service (NHS) and private sector, each with entirely different provision and experience of supervision, dependent on the supervisors and their style. I have also supervised others and early in my career enjoyed developing my skills through supervision training and a course in counselling skills for SLTs. In my NHS roles I had moved from very practical, problem-solving professional supervision with a lead therapist, to more management-focused meetings and I became aware of the loss of opportunity to reflect and develop in my practice, both as a clinician and as a supervisor. I had been fortunate to participate in peer support groups that varied in size, formality, and context in the NHS and private sector. Although these groups were useful, they did not allow me to reflect as deeply as I wanted to. My transition to independent practice happened gradually, initially overlapping with my NHS role, eventually settling with a 'portfolio' of roles comprising lone working and teamwork. Although I only had a few independent clients at first, I wanted to prioritise professional supervision. I sought out a supervisor who I felt met my needs, being both nurturing and very experienced in supervision. This one-to-one relationship is ongoing and has been invaluable as I navigate through my own individual career. Since then, I have started a new one-to-one supervision relationship with a separate supervisor I have known for some years. She is respected in my clinical field and we agreed that this supervision would focus more on clinical formulation and sharing ideas.

I had never experienced peer group supervision and, when Claire and Mary approached me, I was not entirely sure what I was signing up for. Nevertheless, I thought this opportunity was too good to miss. I value sharing clinical experiences with two SLTs who I have known for years but do not work with and was intrigued to engage with supervision that was not one-to-one. As time has passed and we have had more sessions, and worked through developing our triad, I have realised that peer group supervision is much more than that; there is real joy and benefit in talking with colleagues with similar social and cultural backgrounds, training, time in practice and shared values.

Setting up our peer group

At the outset, Claire and Mary talked about values and wishes for this peer supervision group.

We made a positive choice to form a group with therapists who were practising in the same specialism so that we could enhance our clinical practice with people who have a deep, personal experience of the challenging field of acquired brain injury (ABI) rehabilitation.

Drawing on our experience in advanced supervision training was an important foundation. We had benefitted from live supervision practice and agreed that we would adopt this kind of practice and reflection as part of our peer group supervision. To create this possibility, we needed at least three people in our group. Shohet & Hawkins (2012) suggest that a peer group should be no more than seven people to allow adequate time for group members to receive supervision, but we decided that an even smaller group would allow for a more manageable process and simpler scheduling, whilst we learnt about peer group supervision.

Once Kate had accepted our invitation to join the group, our focus turned to contracting how we would work together.

Our group formed during the pandemic, so we could only meet virtually, but, as restrictions lifted, we agreed that our preference was face-to-face meetings. Whilst we continue to use virtual meeting spaces when there are time pressures, ideally, we meet in person. We continue to explore the best locations for meeting, seeking venues that provide a confidential and cost-effective space to meet.

Contracting

Administrative and relational contracting

Drawing on our experience as one-to-one supervisors, we applied contracting to the supervision triad. We discussed and agreed operational aspects of contracting, such as confidentiality, allocation of time and frequency of sessions.

ABI is a small specialism, so we have known each other for many years, but we found it helpful to share stories of studying and working together to establish a current understanding of each other's careers, connections and work contexts. In this way we were able to note any potential conflicts of interest and establish appropriate boundaries and processes for handling them.

We have spoken openly with each other about our different experiences of supervision, which helps us to understand our individual needs. We have all supervised many colleagues and have similar clinical experience but in one conversation we noted that one member had received less current training in supervision. Consequently, we spoke about some supervisor skills more explicitly to ensure that we were all developing a common understanding of our processes.

In peer group supervision it is important to pay attention to multiway contracting so that everyone feels safe and can be open and honest. In a one-to-one supervisory relationship, the supervisee makes a number of decisions about their supervision needs with support from the supervisor. When two or more people are involved in peer group supervision, they each bring individual needs and a discussion around compatibility and compromise may be necessary. For example, we had established the idea of live supervision with feedback in the triad as a core function of the group, but when we became aware of differing levels of supervision training and practice, we gave more time to discussing how live supervision would work and phasing in this practice so that everyone felt comfortable engaging.

Ongoing contracting during each session

The relational aspects of contracting continue to emerge as we meet, which illustrates the importance of allowing time not only to set the tone for the meeting but also leaving time at the end to reflect on the process and suggest changes.

After a couple of sessions, we reflected on our tendency to settle into a pattern of peer support rather than supervision because we were discussing current topics in speech and language therapy and sharing our thoughts and feelings about work life. Each of us value the peer support that we receive through work-based relationships and recognise these relationships are essential for wellbeing in the workplace. We agreed that whilst we would continue to start our sessions with some peer support, we would also pay attention to beginning supervision more intentionally. In practice, this means we set time aside for an initial 'check in' to share important things that are happening in our lives. During this phase, we are in fact gauging mood and energy, as well as deciding what we might be bringing into this supervisory

221

space. It gives each of us a few moments to connect with each other and be intentional about entering the supervisory space. At first, it was helpful to set a timer to bring an end to this part of the supervision but over time, the move into supervision occurs more subtly with one member inviting topics for discussion. Referring to a model, such as the CLEAR supervision model (Hawkins & Smith, 2006), can help to maintain a focus on professional supervision rather than support.

We share the topics we want to discuss and allocate time for each person to receive supervision. Initially we did not choose a lead supervisor but jointly supervised. We noticed that this could set up a distracting contrast between supervision styles, so find it more helpful to identify a lead supervisor, especially if one member is best placed to supervise a particular topic or type of discussion. This natural evolution has allowed us to gradually introduce the idea of identifying the roles and creating a space for live supervision.

To facilitate the development of the group and ensure we are all receiving the supervision we need, we leave 10–15 minutes at the end of each session to reflect on this process and make changes as required.

Benefits of peer group supervision

Together we have applied our knowledge of supervision to a new context and, through contracting and with a shared value set, we have created a safe and trusting space conducive to skill development.

Developing supervisor skills

The qualities needed to supervise in a peer supervision group build on those used in one-to-one professional supervision.

We acknowledge that we each bring different styles of supervising to our group, so it has become a natural setting to model and experience different styles of supervision. One such contrast might be asking questions as opposed to leaving silence for reflection. We make time for discussion and explore together how one style differs from the other and what benefits it brings to the supervisee. We can also allocate time to practise leaving space, if desired.

Sometimes, one peer might employ a supervision technique unfamiliar to the other two. Previously, one peer shared an example of working creatively in supervision; once she had asked a supervisee to share a piece of music that expressed their feelings about a topic. This raised a new creative idea for the other two to explore. We discussed how we could adopt this in our peer supervision group and encouraged and inspired each other to try this new idea in other supervisory settings. It has been confidence-building to explore new techniques together before taking them back into practice as a one-to-one supervisor.

Listening skills are essential for a supervisor. When we co-supervise, listening skills can be honed. This allows the two supervisors to be synchronous and read how the other supervisor is facilitating and responding. Without these skills, sessions can become a little chaotic and potentially distract from the needs of the supervisee.

Building on the live supervision we experienced in our supervision training; we are exploring how we use this format to develop our supervisory skills. Each peer takes a different role, i.e. supervisor, supervisee and observer. During the supervision the observer listens and takes notes for feedback. After the supervision the observer gives feedback at the meta level, offering tentative observations about what was happening with the process of supervision, rather than the clinical discussion. This felt daunting at first but as trust developed, constructive feedback has been extremely beneficial. The observer might note a communication pattern that seems helpful or unhelpful. They may make alternative suggestions about communication style, such as using a more reflective approach or a type of question that might have allowed the supervisee to take a deeper dive into the topic. In this way, in any discussion there is a development opportunity for both the supervisor and supervisee.

We have discovered that peer group supervision is a wonderful environment in which to develop supervisor skills, whatever the nature or starting level of experience we each had as supervisors. We now feel comfortable reflecting on our skills and are becoming increasingly open to talking about areas for skill development, particularly as we observe the principle of being non-judgemental.

Developing supervisee skills and responsibilities

Time is often pressured so it is essential to prepare before each session, i.e. bringing a question or describing a clinical issue concisely, trusting in the skill of the supervisor to use their skills to facilitate the supervisee to explore the topic at hand.

Developing and enriching clinical skills

In our peer supervision group, we are enjoying the benefits of being at a similar stage of our career and working in related clinical areas. The nature of our supervisory relationship, in which we have equal roles within the group, affords a particular type of reciprocal conversation without hierarchy. This is further supported by the fact we do not work together within a departmental structure. However, we think this could also happen within a department when peers approach a peer supervision group arrangement with this attitude of equality. From this perspective, we are well placed to share creative ideas, remind each other of an area of clinical practice that one of us might be more familiar with and encourage each other to find ways together of embedding the evidence base into our practice. As with any form of professional supervision, we aim to nurture existing knowledge in each other rather than give instruction.

Throughout our careers, we can lose confidence from time to time, which can make us feel that there are things we should know but need to ask about. We have noticed it can feel more comfortable to bring these questions to peer group supervision rather than one-to-one because there is no hierarchy. A positive example of this involved one peer bringing a question about adapting conversation partner training (CPT) to address the complexities of support worker (SW) dynamics with a client. The questions felt basic to the therapist but, by acknowledging this and sharing anyway, her peers, who also adapt CPT, were able to facilitate a reflective conversation separating the issues pertaining to CPT and the dynamics as well as share positive examples of CPT from their own experience. This had a restorative impact on the peer with the question, leaving her feeling empowered.

In our peer supervision group, we are all specialists in the field of neurorehabilitation but work in different contexts. We benefit from a common understanding of the challenges of working in this specialism but develop our clinical thinking together because we each approach our work with a slightly different perspective. The outcome of our conversations can be a client-focused intervention that is more than a sum of the parts we each contributed.

Feedback in this context can be incredibly valuable and reassuring because it comes from peers. We have also identified that we can feed off each other's enthusiasm and passion, which leads to a renewed energy for our work and a sense of feeling valued for what we do.

Some surprising outcomes

Meeting together over three years has taught us a lot about the benefits of peer group supervision, including some that were unexpected. Personal commitment to professional supervision comes with both financial and time cost, so there is a practical benefit to peer group supervision; in that it can provide a cost-efficient way to receive additional supervision.

Our meetings are 1.5 hours, divided into a check-in, supervision time (approximately 20 minutes each) and process time. You might assume that this reduces the depth of supervision in any given session. Whilst we are flexible according to everyone's needs and might focus on one or two peers to allow more supervision time, we have also discovered that when one peer raises a topic for discussion, everyone learns something new. A recent example is when one of us raised the topic of transcription. This provoked an interest in the topic for another peer and sparked a new avenue of exploration with multiple perspectives, encouraging that person to go away and consider how transcription could be of value in her practice. Such vicarious learning does not happen in one-to-one supervision because there is no-one extra to witness the conversation. In a peer supervision group, you are exposed to a wider variety of questions by virtue of having more people in the group.

We have all noticed that following a peer group supervision session where one participant has raised a topic for discussion, the others find themselves reflecting on and relating those reflections to their own work life.

Considering the benefits of virtual vs. in-person peer group supervision

We started to meet as a group during the Covid pandemic at a time when it was only possible to meet virtually. Although we were already aware of the use of virtual interfaces in speech and language therapy practice and supervision, the Covid-19 pandemic hastened our take up and enabled us to consider setting up our group even when we could not see each other in person.

Meeting online helped us to focus on the intention of supervision rather than support as the format is more formal. Research suggests that the communication style of peers will also differ significantly in a virtual meeting. We have noted this ourselves and agree with Rousmaniere (2014), who cited studies of supervision dyads which showed better preparation for and reduced inhibition in virtual meetings, facilitating more forthcoming discussions.

We have found that even though we work reasonably close to each other geographically, the use of online meetings can help us maintain regular supervision sessions, especially when we are busy. We also text or email each other between face-to-face meetings, with brief queries. We think that this professional support is possible because of the relationships we have already built in our face-to-face peer group supervision meetings.

Although it is our preference to meet face-to-face, there are wider applications of this online format beyond the pandemic. Online supervision is a really important tool to consider if you do not live in a populous area as it opens up opportunities to develop peer group supervision with people over wider geographical areas. We have also considered how the accessibility and flexibility of online communication would allow for a peer supervision group to form across counties, countries and even continents, enabling us to meet with peers across the globe and enrich our discussions and learning. If this is something that you choose to explore, there might be some issues to consider, such as accounting for different international guidelines and legislation that inform discussion and cultural differences affecting each participant's understanding of the issues brought (Rousmaniere, 2014).

When to engage in peer group supervision

As supervisors, we have noticed that requests for supervision have become more nuanced recently as the interest and understanding of professional supervision deepens across the profession. Typically, enquirers state that they want to attend to one area of practice over another or receive 'supervision of supervision'. There seems to be a greater awareness of the range of possibilities for professional supervision and we would suggest foregrounding peer group supervision as a valuable option.

In our experience combining the benefits of peer group supervision with those of one-to-one professional supervision in particular clinical areas, at specific times, alongside peer support in an ever-evolving mix has been the most rewarding.

We recommend that any newly qualified SLT engages in one-to-one professional supervision as stipulated in the RCSLT 2017 guidelines, however, also envisage that peer group supervision could be a useful complement. That said, each of us had attended at least basic level supervision training before entering a peer group supervision group. This training provided us with essential foundation skills in supervision theory, understanding our supervisee role, supervisor skills and processes, such as contracting with each other. Without this training, it might be more challenging to set up a peer supervision group and one risk would be falling into peer support rather than supervision.

Concluding thoughts

Embarking on peer group supervision together was as much about experiencing a different form of supervision when discussing clinical topics as creating a space to practice supervision skills. Our collective experience has convinced us that peer group supervision is not a luxury but a form of supervision that will remain an important part of our supervision arrangements going forward.

Our peer supervision group processes have evolved over time as we openly discuss our experience and ways in which we would like to develop our supervisory relationship with each other. We have learnt that whilst all forms of supervision have the common aim of providing a safe space to discuss work related issues, the way we receive supervision varies in each setting. Peer group supervision provides a unique space both for support and practice as supervisors and clinicians.

For us, our group is enriching because we are all working in the same specialism. However, a peer supervision group could be formed in a different way and for different reasons. We have discussed how we represent a stereotypical SLT group of white women, and the limitations of peer group supervision with therapists from the same background or culture. A peer supervision group could usefully be set up with a more diverse range of practitioners i.e. across cultures and/or professions. According to Hawkins and Shohet (2012), this provides a breadth of life experience and 'empathic range' that will further enhance practice.

When meeting as a peer group for supervision, we have noticed that the group dynamic comes into focus and without a designated supervisor (as in group supervision) each peer takes responsibility to observe, reflect and support the dynamic for a positive outcome for all. By working together, the group can become increasingly beneficial to each member of the group.

Whatever your reason for setting up a peer supervision group and whatever stage of your career, there are some key decisions to make and conversations to be had. Being clear about what you want from the group and why will inform this process. The more open you are about your needs and pay attention to the needs of others, with reference to the summary below, the more likely you will benefit from a sustainable, enriching peer group supervisory experience.

Group members and size

- The reciprocity of peer group supervision is different to a one-to-one supervisor/supervisee relationship, so choose peers to match your needs; look for peers through your workplace, local therapy team, Clinical Excellence Networks or training courses
- If face-to-face supervision is important to you, look locally
- Ask your one-to-one supervisor to recommend potential peers that could be a good fit
- Once you have started to gather a group, discuss together the optimum group size

Contracting

- Include frequency and length of sessions, confidentiality and how you set agendas in your administrative contract
- Decide on suitable locations, including virtual options and consider the impact these might have on the supervisory process
- Consider the balance of taking on the supervisor and supervisee role and how to switch from one role to another
- Protect processing time at the end of each session to pay attention to the supervisor's skills as well as the supervisee's experience
- Consider participants' history, views and preferences, for example, the supervision style requested by the supervisee. Doing so will benefit the group by fostering a more open and supportive space
- Discuss what to do if conflict arises or anyone is uncomfortable within the group; awareness of any conflicts of interest or power dynamics in the supervision group is essential
- Maintain boundaries i.e. to ensure that supervision within the group does not shift into providing therapy to one of the members
- Review the contract regularly because the extent to which each member benefits from peer group supervision may shift over time. It is important

that people feel they can leave the group if it does not meet their needs, or their commitments have changed whilst maintaining a positive relationship with the other members

We hope that reading about our experience of peer group supervision has inspired you and provides useful guidance to consider peer group supervision in the future.

References

Hawkins, P. and Smith, N. (2006) *Coaching, Mentoring and Organisational Consultancy: Supervision and Development.* Maidenhead: Open University Press.

Hawkins, P. and Shohet, R. (2012) *Supervision in the Helping Professions,* 4th edn. UK: McGraw-Hill Education.

RCSLT (2017) *Information on Supervision.* Available online at: www.rcslt.org/wp-content/uploads/media/docs/delivering-quality-services/infomation-on-supervision.pdf [Last accessed: December 2023].

Kelly, G. A. (1955/1991) *The Psychology of Personal Constructs.* London: Routledge.

Proctor, B. (1986) Supervision: A cooperative exercise in accountability. In M. Marken and M. Payne (eds), *Enabling and Ensuring: Supervision in Practice.* Leicester: National Youth Bureau Council for Education.

Rousmaniere, T. (2014). Using technology to enhance clinical supervision and training. In C. E. Watkins, Jr. and D. L. Milne (eds), *The Wiley International Handbook of Clinical Supervision,* 204–237. Wiley Blackwell.

Going It Alone

18

Being a Supervisee and Supervisor in Independent Practice (and what I have learnt in the process about being human)

Rachel Barton

I worked as a Speech and Language Therapist (SLT) in the UK National Health Service (NHS) for the first 22 years of my professional life. What kept me going in the early years of my career was the people I worked with. As well as having supportive colleagues, I had an excellent supervisor who listened to my concerns, encouraged me to problem solve, and made changes to alleviate the stress where she could. I came to realise that whilst our working context can be far from ideal, the support mechanisms we have in place can make the difference between survival and burnout.

Despite the frustrations of restructures, growing demands, and dwindling resources, my NHS career was a time of professional growth. Key to this was a robust group supervision system introduced by a forward-thinking service manager. All staff were trained in the value, purpose, and skills of supervision as well as a further eight SLTs being trained as group facilitators. Time for supervision was prioritised and attendance was compulsory. The system worked well for many years and provided hours of supervision for the team.

Stepping out of the NHS and into independent practice was not an easy decision. There are many advantages to being in the NHS including working with and learning from colleagues, access to specialists, a predictable and regular income, a good pension, and the knowledge that the service is available for all. Despite this, six years on, I have no regrets. It is reassuring to be working under the same Health and Care Professions Council (HCPC) standards (2023) as the NHS, but with the freedom that comes with working

DOI: 10.4324/9781003301141-18

for myself. Nevertheless, independent practice comes with its own set of challenges and regular supervision remains an essential part of ensuring I deliver a safe, high-quality service whilst also maintaining a good quality of life outside work.

This chapter encompasses my experience and learning from being both a supervisee and supervisor within independent practice. Many of these themes may also be pertinent to those working in other contexts both within and outside of the UK.

Being a supervisee in independent practice

In the UK, the supervision requirements of registering and professional bodies are clear. The HCPC standards of proficiency for SLTs state that registrants must, 'understand the need for active participation in training, supervision and mentoring in supporting high standards of practice, and personal and professional conduct, and the importance of demonstrating this in practice' (HCPC 2023). Similarly, the Royal College of Speech and Language Therapists (RCSLT) has firm guidance, 'Supervision is an essential component of a good quality speech and language therapy service that is able to identify and manage risk. This is the case for all SLTs, including those practising independently or employed in other contexts' (RCSLT 2017). In addition, RCSLT state, 'Failure to access appropriate supervision may affect the indemnity insurance that SLTs have as part of their RCSLT membership'. Sixty to ninety minutes of professional supervision every four to six weeks is RCSLT's recommendation for experienced SLTs.

With this in mind, getting supervision in place was one of the first actions I took when starting independent work. I work alone for a large proportion of my week with little contact with other SLTs and so having regular supervision with someone who understands my work context is vital. When new situations relating to clinical work, professional issues or personal skills arise I am reassured that I will be able to discuss these in depth with my supervisor. This process helps me to ensure I am practising in a safe, ethical, and evidence-based way. In supervision there is always something to learn, some insight to gain, or something to offload which leaves me feeling lighter. Admittedly there is a cost pressure when self-employed; as well as paying for the service, I am forgoing an opportunity to do paid work of my own. However, when supervision works optimally – improving the quality of my service – it is of benefit to me, my clients, and my business in the long-term (as satisfied clients may speak positively about their experiences to others).

In addition to supervision, finding colleagues to link up with in less formal arrangements has been an important part of setting up a wider professional support network. The generous sharing of knowledge, ideas, and support within the independent speech and language therapy community in the UK has been fundamental to maintaining both my professional development and mental wellbeing.

Finding a supervisor

As an independent SLT I had freedom of choice when selecting a supervisor. In the UK there are many places to start looking including local networks of SLTs, the Association of Speech and Language Therapists in Independent Practice (ASLTIP), and wider internet searches. These searches brought up lists of SLTs who were offering supervision but did not guarantee that the SLT had the appropriate skills or training (the role of 'Supervisor' is not protected in the same way that 'Speech and Language Therapist' is). Consequently, it was up to me to satisfy myself that a prospective supervisor had the skills I was looking for. I found it helpful to hear about a person's journey to becoming a supervisor and the approaches they advocated. Whilst an initial conversation was different from a supervision session, it did give some insight into how in tune we were with each other and whether it felt like a relationship worth exploring. In the past I have gained more in supervision when supervisors have taken a supervisee-led approach, helping me to work through problems to find my own solutions. I therefore looked for someone who showed an appreciation for this facilitative style of supervision.

Independent practice supervision involves familiar topics such as clinical discussion, relationships with clients, carers or other professionals, decisions around discharge, and responding to changes in the evidence base. In addition, topics may include the challenges of running a business, our relationship with money, setting boundaries, and preventing professional isolation. For this reason, I looked for a supervisor who had experience in the independent sector. Whilst not essential, I felt it would be helpful to have some shared experience of navigating the business world. In terms of clinical experience, it was useful to know what a supervisor's specific interests and areas of clinical expertise were, but I was more concerned to find a supervisor that I felt comfortable with rather than an exact clinical match. In addition to individual and group supervision for my clinical work I arranged regular supervision for my supervisory work. Seeking different supervision arrangements has been a helpful way of ensuring that all my supervision needs are met.

Becoming a supervisor in independent practice

A significant part of my independent work is offering professional supervision to independent SLTs across the UK. It is extremely fulfilling work and I feel privileged to be invited into other therapists' working lives. I continue to spend half of my week involved in clinical work which helps me to feel in touch with many of the issues and experiences supervisees bring to supervision.

For anyone considering offering supervision, there is a growing demand for supervisors within the independent community. An increasing number of UK SLTs are now working independently in a self-employed capacity, some of whom belong to ASLTIP. The organisation has seen a steady rise in membership now standing at more than 1,600 members (a 68% increase in the last 12 years). There are also opportunities to supervise SLTs employed by schools or charities where professional supervision is contracted externally.

Whether you have a supervision background within your organisation and are looking to use those skills in the independent world or you are coming to the role of a supervisor for the first time, there are a range of areas to consider when developing a robust supervision offer. Reflecting on my experiences, these are the actions that I believe have helped me to build a successful supervision practice:

Reading and research

- Keeping abreast of the evidence base, new developments, and current debates in speech and language therapy
- Keeping a record of interesting articles, books, videos, podcasts and research papers to share

233

Training and development

- Accessing regular supervision for my own clinical and supervisory practice
- Accessing regular training for supervision and related skills (suggested courses at the end of this chapter)

Attracting business

- Dedicating website space for information about my supervision services
- Engaging with forums and social media to join debates, share knowledge and experience, or offer guidance in a professional and thoughtful manner when it is asked for

Clear information

- Providing an information pack to prospective supervisees describing my background, training, supervision approach, and boundaries as well clarifying record keeping procedures and confidentiality

Flexibility

- Offering face-to-face, telephone and online supervision
- Varying length and frequency of sessions to suit each supervisee's needs
- Regularly reviewing the process to ensure it is meeting supervisees' needs

Safe space

- Providing a confidential, non-judgemental, relaxed space where supervisees can express themselves authentically

The supervisory process in independent practice

Whether you are reading this as a supervisee or supervisor, the following insights relate to my experience of how the relationship between these two roles might develop over time.

The initial supervision meeting

I enjoy hearing supervisees recount their careers to date in our first meeting; it can be both illuminating and validating for the therapist. I share information about my own journey and interests as well as making time to explore a supervisee's past experiences of supervision and hopes for the future. We discuss expectations of supervision, explore what other support mechanisms are in place, how we will work together, and what the boundaries will be (see 'Contracting' below). We then spend time exploring an issue the supervisee brings to start the process of supervision.

It is important from the outset to be clear about a supervisor's duty to raise a concern to HCPC if issues around unsafe or unethical practice emerge and are not adequately dealt with. I also explain that whilst I can support supervisees with issues relating to their wellbeing, if a person's needs are beyond my skills and remit, I may suggest accessing a counsellor or other avenues of support.

Contracting

Negotiating a supervision contract is an essential part of developing an effective and safe supervision relationship. We commonly see this practice in other professions (such as counselling or psychotherapy) where the relationship between client and therapist is key to the intended work being effective. As Cassedy (2010) comments, the term 'contract' may be off-putting to some and therefore the term 'working agreement' is sometimes used. In either case, this is a formalisation of the way a supervisee and I agree to work together (with the potential to make changes as the relationship evolves). The supervision contract creates a shared understanding of our purpose and process and helps to prevent difficulties occurring down the line. It can act as reassurance to supervisees of my integrity, adherence to professional standards, and commitment to providing a quality and bespoke service.

Within an organisation there may be standard templates for developing contracts. As an independent supervisor I have developed my own to fit with RCSLT and HCPC guidance, as well as aligning with my own values and ideas. I found this to be a beneficial process to go through as it challenged me to think deeply about my boundaries and my approach. It is also vital when supervising in independent practice that both parties understand the autonomy of the supervisee. Whilst a supervisor can guide, enable, and share information, the decisions that the supervisee makes in relation to their practice must always be their own.

The following topics might be included in a contract; these can be divided into 'administrative' and 'relational' aspects of the supervision process.

Administrative aspects of supervision:

- Frequency and length of sessions
- The format of sessions
- Punctuality and time keeping
- Location of meetings and rules around privacy (including online sessions)
- Dealing with disturbances and setting boundaries around distractions such as phones
- Cancellation and fees
- Areas for discussion e.g. clinical, professional, business, supervisory practice, wellbeing
- Confidentiality and the circumstances under which this may be broken
- A clear process for dealing with concerns e.g. unsafe, or unethical practice
- Record keeping; what the supervisor will make a record of and how, what the supervisee is responsible for recording in line with HCPC standards, and how the supervisee will link this to their professional development log

Relational aspects of supervision:

- The roles and responsibilities of supervisor and supervisee
- The supervisee's career history, past experiences of supervision and hopes for this supervision arrangement
- Potential conflicts of interest

- The supervisor's philosophy and approach to supervision
- Supervisee preferences for questioning and coaching styles
- Areas of strength and areas for development that the supervisee is already aware of
- Key themes related to past practice that might arise in sessions
- Needs and preferences specific to individual identity such as culture, neurodiversity, race, or gender
- Relevant personal information that may affect the supervisee e.g. family or health circumstances
- The process for reviewing the supervision

In line with ASLTIP guidelines (2022), once discussed I write up the contract which can then be mutually signed as a record of the agreement.

Reviewing the contract and supervision process

A supervisee's needs may change over time and hence the importance of regularly reviewing the contract to ensure it remains relevant. This may involve minor adjustments through ongoing discussion or a more formal review. I tend to review the supervision process after a year of working together although the timing of this can be flexible and negotiated with each supervisee. It is an opportunity to reflect on the benefits of supervision, what the supervisee has learnt, and what they would like to change moving forward. Changes may relate to the length or regularity of sessions, hopes for how the supervisory relationship will develop, or how the supervisee would like to approach future sessions.

I also ask supervisees about their key 'take-aways' at the end of each session. This may be an intended action, new knowledge that has been gained, or something a supervisee has learned about themselves.

Questioning techniques

As the SLTs I supervise are autonomous professionals, my central aim is to support individuals to find their own answers wherever possible. A key skill of the supervisor lies in knowing what questions to ask and when to ask to them. For supervisors coming from a background of management supervision, where advising and information giving is a necessary part of the role,

Authoritative Interventions	Facilitative Interventions
Prescriptive	Cathartic
Informative	Catalytic
Confronting	Supportive

Figure 18.1 Heron's Six Categories of Intervention Model (2001)

a transition to this kind of professional supervision can present challenges. However committed one is to providing a place of reflection and facilitation, it can sometimes be hard to suppress the urge to give answers. Taking time to reflect on my questioning style has helped me to constantly hone my facilitation skills.

John Heron's Six Categories of Intervention Model (2001) has formed the basis of my supervision practice over the last 20 years (as well as often being drawn upon in conversations with clients, professionals, friends, and family). It is an ideal framework for firstly identifying a person's position with a presenting issue and secondly the support they might need to move forward. Whilst Heron originally developed this with counselling in mind, he encouraged its wider use in health, social care, education, and business. This model was used extensively in my NHS supervision and has proved equally effective in my independent work.

Heron defines six types of interventions that can be offered when discussing an issue (see Figure 18.1). These are subdivided into 'authoritative' and 'facilitative' interventions.

'Authoritative' includes *prescriptive interventions* e.g. 'I would advise you to contact the safeguarding lead' and *informative interventions* e.g. 'There is an excellent article about this new approach in . . .'. It also includes *confronting interventions* which seek to support the supervisee to challenge attitudes, beliefs, or behaviours that may be preventing them from moving forward with an issue e.g. 'Is there another way of looking at this?'

'Facilitative' interventions are less directive and include *cathartic interventions* which are designed to allow expression of emotions, *catalytic interventions* which aim to elicit problem solving e.g., 'What are your options?' and *supportive interventions* which seek to affirm the worth and value of the supervisee e.g., 'It sounds like you handled that with great care'.

When considering which interventions to use Cassedy (2010, p. 107) explains, 'While none is better than the others, attention needs to be given to which are more appropriate for supervision and the service you are providing to the supervisee'. In the context of independent supervision, I use various interventions, although prescriptive interventions are very rare. Typically, these may be used to advise a supervisee that an issue they have brought should be taken elsewhere e.g. safeguarding, insurance, or legal questions. Supervisees who are 'stuck' with an issue may need cathartic interventions to support the expression of an emotion or confronting interventions to observe a limiting belief or attitude. I highly recommend exploring this model in more depth as a way of developing a supervisee-led approach.

Supporting difference and personal growth

Difference comes in all forms including personality, gender, race, disability, culture, age, sexual orientation, socio-economic status, neurodiversity, and intersectionality. Supervision is a safe space where difference can be acknowledged, valued, and celebrated in the work context. Therapists can examine which aspects of themselves bring greater insight to their work and which aspects bring them personal challenge.

An advantage of being self-employed is that it presents SLTs with the opportunity to develop practice in ways that align more closely with who they are. I often meet SLTs who have found that working in a large organisation creates barriers to being their authentic selves in their work. Independent practice provides more flexibility for SLTs to develop their role and service around their own strengths, values, and aspirations. As a supervisor, I support supervisees working through this transition, enabling the SLT to develop their business in a way that embraces and validates their identity. Examples might be an SLT wanting to develop a client base within their own culture, a neurodivergent SLT wanting to develop administrative processes which align with their most effective ways of working, or an SLT towards the end of their working life who wants to pursue a key project to gain closure on their career.

When challenges arise

The contracting process is an effective way of setting initial boundaries, but new issues may arise as a supervision relationship progresses e.g.

239

a supervisee who consistently needs more time. Solutions might include increasing the length of sessions or aiming to discuss less items. Sometimes boundaries around contact in between sessions also need clarifying. If a supervisee has a difficult issue or a complex question outside of supervision, I may offer an interim short session if the matter is urgent or agree to discuss it at our next session.

Although I aim for supervision to be a facilitative process, I do notice the temptation to give advice. Sometimes a supervisee will ask, 'What would you do?' or, 'What do you think?'. Whilst it is sometimes appropriate to answer these questions, if this happens frequently within a supervision relationship I return to Heron's model and challenge myself to find an approach that will enable the supervisee to problem solve more independently.

It is also essential to be prepared for unsafe or unethical practice being revealed and hence the importance of discussing this in the first meeting. Whatever the challenge that arises, having a plan and some clear boundaries helps in addressing the issue in a straightforward, safe, and honest manner.

Common themes in supervision

Whilst there is huge variation in the clinical and professional issues that are brought to supervision, there are some common themes that frequently arise. Often these are linked to the human condition and may root back to the fundamentals of who we are and how we think. Supervision is not the place where healing from all human struggle can be achieved – nor can this be achieved anywhere – but it can be a space for some reflection about what makes each of us human.

In the six years that I have worked in independent practice I have been fortunate to support over 60 supervisees delivering more than 700 hours of supervision. This has provided me with an insight into the common themes that arise for therapists as well as reassuring me that I am not alone in the challenges I encounter. In the remainder of this chapter, I present some initial insights with some suggestions for further learning in the references. Some of these themes are common in all walks of speech and language therapy but many are particularly pertinent to independent practice.

Perfectionism and people pleasing

As an independent SLT I have sometimes felt a need to go above and beyond because people are paying for my service. This, added to an already over-obliging tendency, meant that I spent unpaid time ensuring all parties were happy and everything was completed to a 'perfect' standard.

Being a perfectionist or a people pleaser is not a conscious decision, it is an environmental response and a pattern that develops in childhood. Recognising, exploring, and understanding these traits in my work has helped me to change my behaviours and attitudes. Refraining from spending extra time and money in an attempt to achieve unrealistic standards has saved me from the feelings of resentment and burnout which I have experienced in the past.

In supervision I support therapists to explore these concepts. We discuss whether actions are 'authentic kindness' (where we give to others whilst maintaining clear boundaries and an awareness of our own needs), or 'people pleasing' which involves sacrificing our own needs for the sake of others (Williams, 2021). We talk about aiming for 'healthy striving' (when we focus on making improvements for ourselves) rather than 'perfectionism' which tends to be driven by fears of what others may think (Brown, 2018). Supervisees also reflect on whether the standards they are setting for themselves are realistic and necessary.

Boundaries and saying 'no'

Discussion of boundaries often leads to talk about the mechanisms of self-validation. I have observed that in saying 'yes', I feel seen, valued, and significant. Learning to say 'no' is becoming easier the more I am able to acknowledge my own worth without relying on external validation. Equally challenging in independent practice is the lack of colleagues for ad hoc discussion around setting healthy boundaries. In my days in the NHS, it was common to return to the office and discuss with colleagues whether a particular request from another professional was reasonable or whether staying late to finish a report was a good decision for my wellbeing. In independent practice therapists often wrestle with these dilemmas alone. This acrostic from OurMindfulLife.com (2022) has resonated with many supervisees over the years:

> *Be aware*
> *Of what is*
> *Unacceptable and*
> *Normalise saying no.*
> *Do what is best for you*
> *And know that it's not your*
> *Responsibility to sacrifice*
> *Yourself for others.*

Work life balance

In my independent practice I have no defined hours of work, no job description, and work comes in sporadically. Accepting new referrals is a tricky balance between keeping a manageable workload and not refusing new business in case there is a quiet period ahead. It is easy to feel overwhelmed resulting in working more hours than intended. The need to present myself as having everything under control can also be a pressure. Supervision can be a time to normalise the chaos of everyday life and reflect on priorities. Practical strategies, like switching off technology and taking time out can be helpful, but if definitions of success are not adjusted there is a danger that therapists continue to feel they have failed to attain the utopian balance they aspire to. What success looks like must be redefined as well as what will be 'good enough' both at work and at home.

Procrastination

Procrastination is a common theme that arises in supervision. Being solely responsible for time management in independent practice can be both freeing and challenging. Adopting specific strategies can increase productivity, but a lack of time management skills is rarely the root cause of difficulties getting started with work. Lieberman (2019) explains that procrastination stems from emotional regulation issues when faced with challenging tasks. The act of procrastinating gives temporary relief from the anxiety, insecurity, or boredom a person might be feeling. Unfortunately, the relief quickly fades, and the anxiety returns leading to further procrastination. A vicious cycle ensues resulting in negative self-judgement. Exploring this phenomenon through a non-judgemental lens can help therapists understand that procrastination is simply part of the human condition. Whilst it may feel counterintuitive, practising forgiveness and self-compassion in times of procrastination is the key to tackling this (with perhaps the odd time management strategy thrown in).

Business matters and imposter syndrome

Independent SLTs can be prone to feeling like an imposter, particularly in the business world. Running accounts, completing tax returns, building websites, and creating marketing strategies are not part of an SLT's basic training. Many therapists assume that their caring nature means that they are not naturally gifted in the qualities needed to run a successful business.

Supervision is an ideal place to contemplate some more challenging aspects of business such as writing terms and conditions, creating contracts, understanding changes in the law, or navigating through a global crisis. The COVID-19 pandemic was an impressive illustration of the responsiveness of the independent workforce, with many SLTs delivering a new version of online therapy within days of going into lockdown. The creativity and problem-solving skills SLTs possess are in fact ideal in developing successful and innovative businesses.

Sharing with a supervisee that imposter syndrome is a widespread phenomenon, experienced by many including myself, often helps to normalise these feelings. It is also helpful to highlight that imposter syndrome is commonly experienced by high achieving, competent people and so more likely a sign of conscientiousness than incompetence (Cox, 2018).

Money

Knowing what to charge and how to discuss this with clients was something I initially found daunting. Many SLTs also have a feeling of unease when asking for payment. This may be related to background, culture, feelings of worth, and empathy for families managing in today's financial climate.

Frank discussion in supervision about feelings around money can help to approach this in a fair way for both the therapist and client. I have found it helpful to reflect on the time and money I have invested in training and professional development, the unique personal skills I have to offer, the knowledge and experience I bring to the role, and a family's autonomy in choosing to pay me for these. An hourly rate is often reflective of much more than one hour's work and charging for both contact and non-contact work is equally justified. I remind myself that in employed roles I had holiday and sick pay, a pension, and regular working hours with a predictable income. As I sacrifice these benefits for the freedom and flexibility of working for myself, it is important I adequately compensate myself for the work that I do. If I truly believe that I am worth the money I am charging, it becomes easier to unapologetically request payment from clients.

Shifts in professional culture and practice

Supervision is the perfect place for SLTs to dig more deeply into attitudes and historical practices and identify potential changes. The recent surge of information in relation to neurodiversity has provided many hours of thoughtful discussion in supervision sessions. Supervision has been a powerful place to work through feelings of defensiveness or guilt when discovering that past practices may have been ineffective or even harmful. Therapists have shared, challenged, and integrated new ideas into their practice combining research, clinical experience, and the lived experience of others. We have discussed research articles or podcasts and reflected on how the learning can be built into our practice.

Supervision is also a place where therapists can admit to not knowing, feeling confused, or needing help or guidance without fear of judgment or professional embarrassment. Acknowledging gaps in knowledge and skills is an essential part of continuing professional development and happens most easily in a safe and confidential space.

Professional isolation

Moving from a busy team to working from home in a one-person business was a considerable change for me. Many SLTs find that they miss the camaraderie and support of colleagues when they make such a move. Supervision is one way to gain contact, but it needs to be part of a wider approach. Support networks can be built through local independent speech and language therapy groups, Clinical Excellence Networks, peer supervision groups and attending training. Social media, when viewed with a critical eye, provides opportunities to become involved in discussions and helps therapists to discover what is developing in the profession within their country and around the world. In supervision, therapists can reflect on the adequacy of their professional support network to avoid the potential difficulties of isolation from peers.

Concluding thoughts

Whilst the fundamental role of supervision is to support quality of clinical practice, therapists cannot do this in isolation from themselves. The difficulties that are encountered at work and the barriers that people face are likely to be reflective of the issues that arise in their lives more generally. Deeper self-exploration and reflection becomes an integral part of supervision. For this reason, it is important that supervisors are sufficiently trained and comfortable with discussing emotions, vulnerabilities, and difficulty. Supervision is not a substitute for counselling or therapy, but it may be the place where the need for this is first recognised and discussed.

The supervision relationships that are formed in independent practice can be long lasting, deeply meaningful and a lifeline for those working in roles isolated from speech and language therapy colleagues. When a safe, confidential, and non-judgmental space is offered, it allows practitioners to be authentic and the issues that have the most meaning for them come to light. The common themes that arise in supervision often lead back to a person's need to value and believe in themself. I see this reflected in myself and the many SLTs that I work with. We do our best work when we believe in ourselves, and we believe in ourselves when we do our best work.

References

Association of Speech and Language Therapists in Independent Practice (2020). *ASL-TIP Guidelines 2020–2021: Supervision*. Available online at: https://asltip.com/members-area/documents/supervision-document/ [Accessed 03 September 2022].

Brown, B. (2018). *The Gifts of Imperfection: Let Go of Who You Think You're Supposed to Be and Embrace Who You Are*. Minnesota, Hazelden.

Cassedy, P. (2010). *First Steps in Clinical Supervision. A Guide for Healthcare Professionals*. Maidenhead, Open University Press.

Health and Care Professions Council (2023). *The Standards of Proficiency for Speech and Language Therapists*. Available online at: www.hcpc-uk.org/stan

dards/standards-of-proficiency/speech-and-language-therapists/ [Accessed 20 October 2023].

Heron, J. (2001). *Helping the Client: A Creative Practical Guide,* 5th edn. London, Sage.

Lieberman, C. (2019). *Why You Procrastinate (It Has Nothing To Do With Self-Control).* Available online at: www.nytimes.com/2019/03/25/smarter-living/why-you-procrastinate-it-has-nothing-to-do-with-self-control.html [Accessed 29 October 2023].

Our Mindful Life (2022). *28 Boundary Quotes to Say No without Feeling Bad.* Available online at: www.ourmindfullife.com/boundary-say-no-quotes/ [Accessed 28 April 2022].

Royal College of Speech and Language Therapists (2017). *Supervision: Information for Speech and Language Therapists.* Available online at: www.rcslt.org/wp-content/uploads/media/docs/delivering-quality-services/supervision-summary-for-speech-and-language-therapists.pdf [Accessed 28 April 2022].

TED-Ed (2018). Elizabeth Cox. *What is imposter syndrome and how can you combat it?* Available online at: www.ted.com/talks/elizabeth_cox_what_is_imposter_syndrome_and_how_can_you_combat_it?language=en#t-167987 [Accessed 28 April 2022].

Williams, P. (2021). *5 Differences Between People Pleasing and Authentic Kindness.* Available online at: https://medium.com/change-your-mind/5-differences-between-people-pleasing-and-authentic-kindness-4b50d31a53f2 [Accessed 28 April 2022].

Suggested courses:

https://intandem.co.uk/courses/

www.citylit.ac.uk/courses/acceptance-and-commitment-therapy-for-speech-and-language-therapists

https://michaelpalincentreforstammering.org/tc-events/solution-focused-brief-therapy-thepalincentre/

https://mindfulnesssussex.co.uk/courses-we-offer.html

www.thelinkcentre.co.uk/courses/the-official-introduction-to-transactional-analysis-ta101/

https://asltip.com/courses/

Looking Back and Looking Forward

Facilitating Robust Supervision Culture and Practice through Training

Sam Simpson and Cathy Sparkes

This chapter is a personal reflection on our journeys over the past twenty years during which we have championed supervision for and on behalf of the speech and language therapy (SLT) profession and beyond. Although considered central to best practice, our experience has shown that training in relation to supervision has been poorly represented in pre-qualification and continuous professional development (CPD) opportunities within SLT nationally. Indeed, Health Education England (2020) acknowledged that 'for many health professionals, career development in clinical knowledge and skills is prioritised over development in [. . .] supervision knowledge and skills'. This chapter tracks our development of a range of supervision training courses since 2006 and reflects on emerging themes and learning points that have positively impacted participant supervision practice. These can be divided as follows: an understanding of professional guidance and access to supervision theory; the importance of shared group learning opportunities; and experiential and creative learning opportunities that support theory into practice.

We hope that our experiences will give some insight into how supervision and practitioner self-care have become a higher priority for organisations, services, and individuals and how understandings of supervision are communicated across our profession. We strongly encourage you, the reader, to take an active role in learning about supervision, the different forms it can take and how it can enrich professional practice and support practitioner wellbeing. We hope this chapter increases your commitment to prioritising yourself in your work through regular access to high quality supervision.

DOI: 10.4324/9781003301141-19

For transparency, we will start by introducing ourselves to provide a clearer insight into the lenses through which we view supervision and supervision training. We have chosen to write predominantly in the first-person plural to maintain a cohesive shared voice. Where our experiences differ, our supervision histories are written in the first-person singular. A further point of language relates to our use of the term supervision. When used in isolation, we use 'supervision' to refer to both managerial and professional supervision. When differentiating between the two, our language use is more specific.

Sam

I entered the profession as a postgraduate in 1995. My career has since taken several twists and turns including working briefly with children under five and their parents; more extensively in adult neurorehabilitation; and for the entirety of my career with adults who stammer, through which I have developed a particular interest in critical disability studies, stammering activism and what stammering can teach us about ourselves and the world. I am also a person-centred counsellor and have worked in this capacity with adolescents and adults in education, the voluntary sector and independent practice since 2009. The person-centred approach is based on the idea that we are all unique and the true experts on ourselves. These central premises underpin my work as a speech and language therapist, counsellor, supervisor and trainer.

Supervision has been a running stitch throughout my career. In 1995 supervision was more established within some NHS Trusts and organisations than others and was a key factor in my choice of workplace. I quickly discovered the centrality of professional supervision to my practice, and I am deeply indebted to the myriad professional supervisors who have since supported me. Professional supervision has offered me a safe, non-judgemental and confidential space to reflect openly and honestly on my personal and professional responses to my work, enabling a greater understanding of my values and my needs. It has been the refuge I have taken moments of uncertainty, frustration, self-doubt, isolation and self-judgement. It is where I have grappled with my career direction, navigated life transitions and celebrated achievements, no matter how small. Professional supervision is the first thing I put in my work diary and the last thing I take out. It keeps me alert to comfort and complacency and facilitates novel practice narratives. As such, professional supervision is instrumental in supporting me to be a reflective, ethical and creative practitioner, supervisor and trainer.

Cathy

I worked as a speech and language therapist from 1986 before retraining and subsequently practising as a personal construct psychology (PCP) counsellor since 2004. My areas of interest and expertise include working with individuals with a neurological condition and their families, supervising a range of allied health professionals (AHP) in public, private and charitable sectors and teaching in areas of supervision, creative counselling skills and PCP.

When I initially entered the SLT profession I found myself in a department where professional supervision was neither offered nor seen as an essential part of professional practice. I was regarded as unusual asking for it. Following a foundation course in PCP, I became aware of the need to prioritise myself and reflect on my work, challenge myself and put that feedback into practice. So, I paid for professional supervision from outside the NHS from a practitioner who was a speech and language therapist and counsellor. Going forward in my career, I did manage to access professional supervision within the NHS as I actively chose to work in organisations whose culture supported high quality supervision. I continue to receive external professional supervision alongside any supervision from within an organisation, as I have always benefitted from a perspective outside my specific work context.

My knowledge and understanding of supervision increased through attending and offering courses, workshops, informal forums, relevant reading, receiving and offering different styles of supervision and creating a service culture which prioritised supervision and self-care. I understand the importance of being in tune with my own core values as a person, as a professional and as a supervisor. These continue to be authenticity, respect, self-awareness, flexibility, investment in myself and the opportunity for experimentation.

Our shared beliefs around supervision

Although we write from diverse supervision histories, we also write from what we share: a fundamental belief that supervision is essential to high quality SLT practice. We continue to observe significant discrepancies in supervision practice within the profession and note that professional supervision is typically accessed less frequently than managerial supervision and professional support. This disparity has motivated us to advocate for robust supervision culture and practice that clearly delineates between managerial supervision, professional supervision and professional support.

We both believe that:

- Professional self-care includes a balance of managerial supervision, professional supervision and professional support
- Regular, quality managerial and professional supervision is a right for all practitioners throughout their careers and needs to be bespoke and flexible to accommodate changes in a therapist's working practice over time
- All supervision provides a safety net for both client and practitioner
- All supervision offers a safe, confidential, and reflective space outside of and linked to practice. Supervision does not happen in a vacuum. It is intricately connected to and informed by practice, the context of the work and learning about practice whether with others or independently
- All supervision is centred in a contracted, confidential and boundaried working relationship characterised by respect and the balance of power, support, and challenge
- Each supervisory arrangement is a unique, negotiated encounter between supervisee and supervisor within the context of the supervisee's work
- Each supervision contract needs to be reviewed regularly, enabling a metaconversation about both the practice of supervision and the supervisory relationship
- Professional supervision is where the sharing of uncertainties, concerns and personal process is welcomed, where mistakes are seen as an integral part of learning and where professional development, clients and ethics are held firmly at the centre of learning. Fundamental to this is the importance of having access to a choice of professional supervisors outside of the management structure, thus promoting safety, consistency, and integrity in the supervisory relationship
- Whilst all professional supervision is learning, not all learning is professional supervision. We consider professional supervision a

central strand of learning about practice, yet distinct from education and counselling

Looking back

Genesis and evolution: An iterative approach to course development

Following the death of Jayne Comins, a speech and language therapist who had championed supervision within the UK SLT profession, we were inspired to build on her legacy and run our first supervision training course in 2006. Our training experience had shown us that many practitioners were not receiving consistent or high quality supervision. Consequently, we were keen to support practitioners to understand their right and professional duty to give themselves a regular space and time to reflect on their work in the form of supervision. We wanted participants to recognise the benefits of this not only for themselves, but for their clients, families and the wider service. We hoped our first one-day supervision course would equip practitioners with the knowledge, skills and confidence to prioritise themselves in their work and foreground their own learning and professional wellbeing.

We were tentative at first, however trusted that our combined supervision practice and teaching experience were robust enough to hold our shared uncertainties. Drawing on our previous experience of running other courses, we involved participants early via pre-course questionnaires to help determine course content and style. This approach mirrored the way we believe that supervision should be offered and received – a collaboration in which both supervisor and supervisee share their knowledge and learning simultaneously: two 'experts' in the room. Listening to participants before, during and after each training was central to the balance of theory, experiential learning opportunities and skills practice included in the courses that we subsequently developed. Each iteration and new course drew directly on our teaching experience and participant feedback. Content was shaped by the dilemmas participants brought to the courses, reflections on their supervision culture and context, our own experiences of SLT and counselling supervision as both supervisees and supervisors and additional supervision training and independent reading.

In addition, we responded to requests for a range of courses to accommodate different levels of knowledge, training and supervision practice experience, geographical locations, types of service and setting (e.g. hospital, community, outreach, education), professional backgrounds (uni- vs. multi-professional groups) and delivery contexts (e.g. external vs. in-house training; in-person vs. online delivery). Over time we have noted several changes in the context and make-up of course participants including a move from:

- Primarily NHS practitioners to more independent practitioners. As sole workers, independent practitioners often find themselves with no supervision structure in place and the need to find appropriate supervision in accordance with the requirements of the Health and Care Professions Council (HCPC). Many independent practices have developed clear supervision structures and include attendance at supervision training as part of their induction process, as have a growing number of NHS Trusts over the years
- Predominantly speech and language therapists to multidisciplinary professionals. We suggest this reflects a greater interest in more integrated training across professions and a possible paucity of quality supervision training within allied health and care professions
- Scheduled courses to a greater number of commissioned courses both with uni- and multi-professional teams (e.g. hospital services, rehabilitation units, community teams, education services). We observe that working regularly with practitioners within the same organisation creates a springboard for sustained change at an individual, team and service level
- Working face-to-face to working online. Take up has significantly increased nationally since the pandemic in 2020 as online courses became more readily accessible and affordable, enabling increased equity of access. We also suspect that Covid-19 has highlighted the importance of practitioner wellbeing for everyone

Changes within the regulatory landscape have also influenced the content and style of our training courses. One key initiative was being commissioned as lead writers for the Royal College of Speech and Language Therapists (RCSLT) Information on Supervision (2017) to raise awareness of personal and organisational responsibility and accountability for supervision.

This guidance has increased practitioners' understanding of the scope and potential of supervision, and empowered them to assert personal, professional, and service needs in relation to high quality supervision and self-care. We are encouraged that the RCSLT (2023) Professional Development Framework positions supervision as a primary means of facilitating learning at all career levels and across all settings. HCPC, through their webpages and 2023 revised guidance, have further reinforced the importance of supervision across all allied health and care professionals: 'Supervision plays a key part in supporting professional development and learning, so it's essential that everyone engages effectively as part of their practice' (HCPC, 2021). Consequently, supervision and practitioner self-care have both become a higher priority for organisations, services, and individuals. We welcome these changes to the regulatory landscape and hope the participant-led insights shared in this chapter can support comprehensive supervision training practices across all AHP professions and health and care pathways.

Over time, a series of Foundation level courses and Advanced Supervision workshops took shape which offer cumulative learning opportunities. Their evolution was ad hoc and experimental. We regularly questioned what we were offering, who we were reaching and how to have a greater impact on individuals, organisations and the profession more widely. Ongoing evaluation was paramount and participant feedback foregrounded the importance of the following key components:

- A balance of personal, experiential and reflective learning opportunities
- Integrating supervision theory into practice
- Defining the supervisee and supervisor roles and responsibilities which underpin robust supervision practice
- Exploring practical frameworks that can be taken forward into diverse workplaces
- Cultivating flexibility and creativity within supervision practice
- Providing a forum for exploring supervision practice concerns and dilemmas
- Embedding the importance of supervisors accessing regular supervision of their own supervision practice
- Networking and building a community of practitioners committed to high quality supervision practice

Core training elements that positively impact supervision practice

We have noticed the following core elements of our training courses that positively impact participant supervision practice are:

- An understanding of professional supervision guidance and access to supervision theory
- Opportunities for shared group learning
- Experiential and creative learning opportunities that support theory into practice

We will elaborate on each of these components in turn.

An understanding of professional supervision guidance and access to supervision theory

One recurrent theme is that practitioners entering our training courses typically lack a reliable understanding of supervision theory and professional guidance, with their supervision practice largely improvised and/or influenced by previous supervision experience. Practitioners typically replicate supervision practice they have found helpful and actively discontinue supervision practice that has been experienced as unhelpful or harmful. We find it striking how pivotal early experiences of supervision as trainees and newly qualified practitioners can be and the central role these experiences take in shaping future understandings, beliefs and attitudes towards supervision.

Being given an opportunity to explore individual and collective definitions of supervision and compare these with the supervision literature enables participants to begin to establish a clearer understanding of what supervision is and is not. This is enhanced by an awareness of professional guidance (RCSLT, 2017; Health Education England, 2020; RCSLT, 2023; HCPC, 2023) which enables a clear distinction to be made between managerial supervision, professional supervision, and professional support. Through the training, participants come to understand that in practice boundaries can often be blurred between managerial and professional supervision when they are not delivered by separate supervisors. Frequently, they identify that managerial supervision is prioritised over professional supervision and that organisational paperwork can drive the supervisory process as opposed to the supervisee. In addition, participants may discover that what they previously considered to be professional supervision is in fact professional support and they are not receiving professional supervision at all.

We have observed that learning the importance of professional supervision in relation to practitioner wellbeing, clinical governance and client safety as well as accountability typically fosters course participants' commitment to it. This is reinforced by an understanding that not accessing professional supervision can lead to defensiveness, rigidity and burnout, all of which directly impacts the supervisee, their clients and the wider service. Through the training courses, participants can acknowledge and explore the personal and professional challenges of their work and the toll that high demand, complex caseloads, working under pressure to increasingly tight deadlines and daily exposure to trauma can take. This invariably leads to a greater focus on prioritising themselves in their work and commitment to accessing regular professional supervision as a means of supporting self-care. This is further consolidated by a knowledge of professional best practice guidance and a clearer understanding of their own responsibilities in terms of ethical practice. An understanding of RCSLT (2017) recommendations regarding the frequency of both managerial and professional supervision offers participants an opportunity to reflect on their current arrangements and the extent to which they are meeting their professional requirements.

Having an opportunity to critique a range of theoretical frameworks that show the evolution of supervision theory since the 1980's and relate these to their own personal experience of supervision builds participant confidence in translating theory into practice. For example, awareness of developmental models of supervision (Stoltenberg & Delworth, 1987; Stoltenberg, McNeil & Delworth, 1998; Hawkins & Shohet, 2012) consolidates the understanding that supervision needs change over time and underlines the importance of flexibility on the part of both the supervisee and the supervisor in the relationship. For example, a practitioner might feel confident and competent in one area of the work and more uncertain in another. These models also encourage practitioners to use supervision to pay attention to specific points of transition in their careers, such as moving up a grade and taking on new roles and responsibilities, moving to a new service, location or area of specialism or returning to work after parental leave, a career break or a bereavement.

Opportunities for shared group learning

As supervision is a relational practice, a group setting is a natural learning environment to develop supervision knowledge, skills, and practice. In our experience, a combination of whole and small group opportunities contributes to the richness of shared learning and reflection.

A central strand throughout the courses is the focus on therapist self-awareness. The courses aim to emulate what is possible in relation to supervision practice, supervisory relationships, and pro-supervision culture through direct engagement with different modes, models, and approaches to supervision as well as teaching, sharing and reflection. Witnessing others engaging in and reflecting on the supervisory process as both supervisees and supervisors creates opportunities to learn from and with each other as well as from us. This balancing and sharing of power within the group again models the dynamics of equity and collaboration intrinsic to effective supervision practice. Opportunities to hear other participants' supervision stories within different organisational structures and to work across disciplines expands participants' understandings of the scope of supervision practice. This breadth of experience supports challenge and therapist self-enquiry alongside honest reflection and conversation, which in turn often leads to a greater willingness to take risks and experiment within and outside of the courses.

We respect different learning styles and levels of experience by providing a range of teaching approaches and levels of training. Within a course we consider personal preferences and try to be responsive to these during the day. Examples of this include inviting people to ask questions, opening up a conversation around a specific dilemma, tailoring discussions to explore a particular challenge, or pairing participants with relevant experience. Across courses, we support practitioners' progress through the training at their own pace and to a level that suits their needs and interests. Some practitioners are keen to explore supervision practice from the perspective of supervisee whereas others prioritise the perspective of supervisor. We offer a range of course options to enable participants to attend individually, as a pair or small group or as a whole team or service. In this way practitioners have the opportunity to learn from and with diverse practitioners either from within or outside their own field on a uni-disciplinary or cross-discipline basis.

Motivation to meet other practitioners interested in supervision and to learn from and with them is a common driver for participants. As an individual practitioner, access to shared group learning fosters a greater sense of connection with and support from a community of therapists committed to robust supervision practice. We encourage ongoing relationships and contact between participants following the courses to further support the learning process. For example, we are aware of course triad groups who have subsequently created regular peer supervision skills practice groups to support ongoing supervisor development. Similarly, one-to-one and peer supervisory relationships have grown out of paired work and discussions. We hope that prioritising supervision and practitioner self-care becomes normalised and consolidated by witnessing others doing the same. Reflecting on the adequacy of current supervision arrangements in a group environment gives practitioners a point of comparison and sense of new possibilities. We have observed this often results in course participants taking greater responsibility in directing their own supervisory arrangements to meet their wants and needs. Signposting supervisor registers/databases further reinforces the importance of choice of supervisor and the value of meeting with several potential candidates in order to make an informed decision about compatibility.

Supervision training for whole teams, single- and multi-professional services and NHS Trusts, whether in-person or online, offers a very different learning environment to attending an external course on an individual basis. Whole team training can act as a catalyst to re-configure and optimise supervision culture and practice across wider services as well as a shared commitment to change. We are encouraged by the visible cultural shifts and increasing dedication to quality supervision practice we have witnessed across both the public and independent sectors in recent years. More therapists, organisations and services are demonstrating commitment to developing embedded supervision structures and practices, greater differentiation between managerial and professional supervision, flexibility and choice of supervisor, and protected time for supervision. One indicator for supervision becoming a higher professional development priority for practitioners and their employers includes greater funding being made available to senior managers/AHP leads to invest in whole team and service training. To support this change, a growing number of supervision champions, working parties and change management processes are being developed to enable ongoing review and evolution over time. This is evidenced by a number of authors in this edition.

Experiential and creative learning opportunities that support theory into practice

> Supervision is a form of experiential learning, of learning from practice. Supervision is reflection-on-action, or indeed reflection-in-action, to result in reflection-for-action.
>
> (Carroll, 2014, p. 16)

Due to the emphasis placed on experiential learning within our courses, it is important to establish clear boundaries, a confidentiality agreement, and any conflicts of interest (e.g. pre-existing or current supervisory or managerial relationships) within the group from the outset of each course. This helps to create safe learning environments where all questions, experiences and uncertainties are valued and can be explored openly and honestly. In this way we set up training group dynamics that prioritise relationships and the centrality of trust, thereby modelling the importance of these within supervision practice.

Course participant feedback consistently affirms how valuable experiential learning opportunities are to integrating and consolidating theoretical understandings as well as developing supervision practice. Examples include paired work practising listening for deeper understanding; unpacking the impact of different questioning styles and extended triad practice enabling each participant to rotate between supervisee, supervisor, and observer. Such varied opportunities to experiment, reflect and gain peer and tutor feedback in a supportive environment builds confidence in being both a supervisee and a supervisor and deepens participants' understanding of core supervision skills, roles, and responsibilities.

Schuck and Wood (2011) advocate the use of creative methods in supervision to link right- and left-hemisphere understandings of practice, thereby facilitating new perspectives, fresh energy and clarity. We give course participants first-hand experience of working with different media, including pen/paper, images, 3D materials such as stones, buttons and everyday objects, as well as working with constellations, the blob tree (Wilson & Long, 2008) and the Pictor technique (King et al., 2013). Integrating creative approaches within our supervision training courses offers a more holistic approach, enabling participants to access their own innate knowledge and personal resources without relying on language.

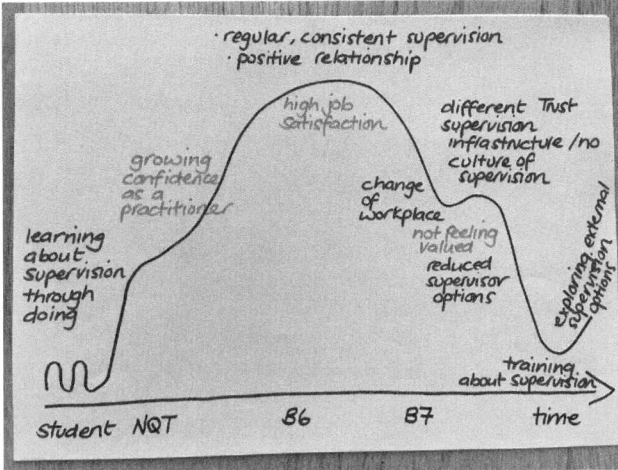

Figure 19.1 Example of a supervision timeline

A creative example designed to mirror the supervisory process in a practical way is the 'supervision timeline' as shown in Figure 19.1. Participants on the first training course are invited to plot out and represent their supervision history as supervisee (and supervisor if relevant) visually through drawing or mind mapping. This vantage point has the potential to open up novel reflections, connections and insights. Subsequent paired discussion makes space to reflect on the nature, regularity and quality of the supervision received, and the relationship between supervision experiences and work enjoyment, career development and preferred supervision style. This activity can be taken directly into practice. For example, in an initial exploratory session, a supervision timeline can support a supervisee and supervisor to explore their respective understandings of supervision. It also enables helpful and unhelpful past supervision experiences to be unpacked to determine potential barriers to the relationship and supervisory process going forward. Being unsure what supervision is and/or having little or no previous experience of it to draw on are barriers that can inhibit people from seeking or engaging actively in supervision.

In subsequent supervisor training courses, we encourage participants to use self-selected items to represent themselves, others and situations

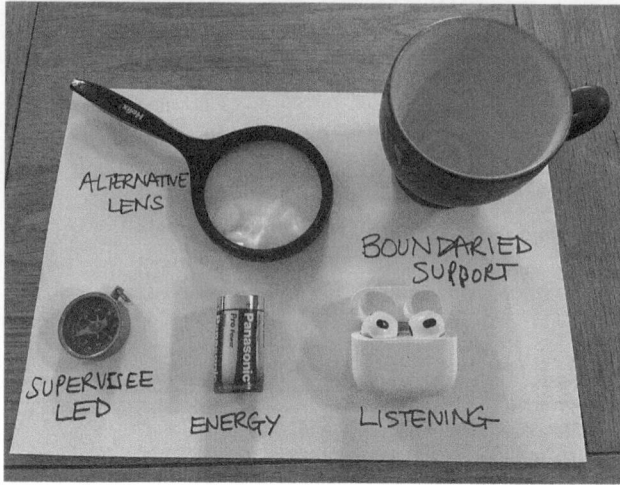

Figure 19.2 Example of objects chosen to support a supervisor elevator pitch

within the supervision arena. For example, inviting participants to select images to represent core values as a supervisor and gain awareness of what informs their supervision practice. Alternatively, choosing a selection of objects around the house to support 'a supervisor elevator pitch' and experiment with speaking to their underlying supervisor philosophy, as shown in Figure 19.2.

Based on the Pictor technique (King *et al.*, 2013), different coloured post-it notes can be used to map similarities and differences in a supervisory relationship as demonstrated in Figure 19.3. This offers a visual means of exploring systems of power and privilege to identify whether these are held implicitly or explicitly and to investigate ways these can inform and support the supervisory process.

Such activities foster dynamic and memorable learning opportunities that build confidence and consolidate new learning. Course participants are regularly surprised at the potential these creative approaches have to reveal fresh insights and open up possibilities regarding themselves and others as well as expand and strengthen their supervision vocabulary. Having directly experienced the benefits, practitioners are then keen to embed these innovative ways of working in their supervision practice.

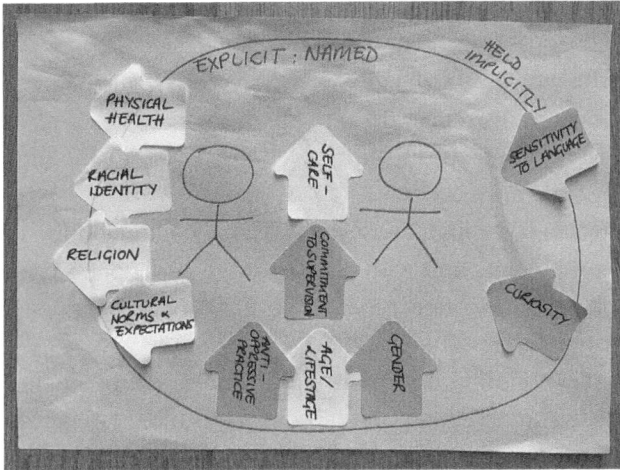

Figure 19.3 Example of a visual map of similarities and differences in a supervisory relationship

In summary: Our learning as a trainers, facilitators and course developers

Writing this chapter has enabled us to reflect deeply on our learning as trainers and course developers. In offering you our insights, we hope to encourage creativity, experimentation and community building in the area of supervision.

Creating and delivering courses is not for the faint-hearted and we have needed to be willing to question ourselves every step of the way. We were our own critics, noticing similar and different aspects of the way each training event transpired. We stayed alert to what participants were drawn to, what they asked for more information about and when they seemed to be fully engaged or less interested. At the end of each course, we would make time to share our own reflections, observations, and evaluations. We considered and amended parts of the course so that each subsequent training day would be more tailored to the feedback going forward. No mean feat in practice as different participants often wanted more or less of particular aspects of the day, so navigating these tensions and contradictions has been challenging at times.

261

As we look back over time, particular high points have been working:

- with small to medium sized groups (i.e. six to 20 participants) to optimise individual learning, reflection and skill development
- across diverse contexts, including NHS Trusts, charitable organisations, and independent practice
- with groups of participants who know each other to mobilise whole team supervision cultures and with groups where participants are unfamiliar with each other to connect them with a growing community of practitioners interested in supervision
- with single discipline and multi-professional groups (including physiotherapists, occupational therapists, psychologists, social workers, doctors, nurses, dietitians, podiatrists, orthoptists, operating department practitioners, headteachers, educators, music therapists, sign language interpreters, administrators, assistants, and technicians across professions)

Through interactions, reading other professions' supervision guidance and the cross-discipline supervision we offer, we have been proactive in seeking to understand the cultures and philosophies of the different professions we have worked with, noticing the diverse lenses through which each might view supervision. Creating regular opportunities to discuss these different constructions and understandings of supervision across professional boundaries has been enlightening for us and participants alike. It has also underscored the importance of establishing a shared understanding of supervision from the outset. This process within the teaching context again parallels initial conversations in a supervisory relationship where both parties need to have a clear understanding of each others' perspective on and experience of supervision.

Looking forward

We recognise that speech and language therapists possess excellent communication skills, including counselling and emotional support skills (such as empathy, listening skills, awareness of different questioning styles) as well as clinical knowledge. However, we observe that at all stages, including transition points between different grades there are inherent assumptions and expectations that therapists step up to the next level and by osmosis develop the requisite skill set to take on the changing role of supervisor. Speech and language therapists are all too frequently required to develop their supervisory skills implicitly without access to ongoing training opportunities through which these skills can be reflected on, reinforced explicitly and consolidated. We are struck by how poorly this contrasts to similar transitions in the field of counselling.

In recent years, there has been a growth in post-qualification supervision training courses for counsellors and psychotherapists with nationally recognised qualifications and accreditation possibilities following the creation of clear professional guidance on core supervisor competencies and training requirements. We would welcome this development within the field of SLT. We envisage nationwide basic supervision training available for junior therapists which would be a prerequisite prior to embarking on the supervision of students and assistants. Intermediate supervision training could then be available to more experienced therapists and clinical specialists making the transition into the supervisor role with newly qualified and less experienced speech and language therapists. Subsequently, advanced supervision training could be open to all managers, team leads, or senior therapists required to supervise staff from multiple professional backgrounds and levels of experience. We strongly believe that a nationally recognised, accredited, and mandatory supervision training programme, like the well-established basic, intermediate, and advanced dysphagia training programmes, would be advantageous. Such a programme would not only recognise the complexity of supervision and the range of skills and roles required of the supervisee and supervisor but would also support the development of more established understandings of supervision practice from which to develop and grow as a profession. Putting supervision on the map in a more sustainable way would not only support a more robust supervision culture within the profession but would also foster stronger supervision infrastructures within services and across organisations. Additionally, we would welcome in-depth supervision training being embedded in university education programmes, as part of work induction programmes and ongoing in-service training as well as investment in ongoing supervision of supervision to support best practice.

Whilst we are encouraged by the growing commitment to quality supervision within the SLT profession, we challenge the culture of complacency and unsatisfactory supervision practice at both the level of the individual and organisation that is still evident in many areas. This will require not only a cultural shift in investing in qualified supervisors and supervision infrastructure, but also a financial commitment to paying for supervision externally if a suitable supervisor is not available within an organisation. Accessibility to a choice of recognised supervisors would be aided by a national supervision register of qualified supervisors, held for example by RCSLT. A true valuing of the role could also lead to recognised consultants in supervision and bespoke posts fostering high quality supervision practice and culture, supported by a National Supervision Clinical Excellence Network and an RCSLT Advisor. Furthermore, ongoing cross-professional collaboration will be needed to ensure supervision practices fully support the supervision needs of developing multi-professional advanced clinical practitioners.

We appreciate this is an ambitious vision for supervision within and beyond the profession going forward. It raises questions about the role of registrant and employer responsibility, how quality assurance will be applied and how variations in supervision practices and understandings across professions can be navigated. However, we believe a greater commitment and investment in AHP supervision training and practice to be integral to maintaining a well-resourced and highly skilled workforce as well as reinforcing public safety. We hope our training courses have helped to sew multiple seeds that over time will germinate and realise this vision in robust and generative ways. Thus, as we picked up the supervision baton from Jayne Comins, we look to pass it on to future generations of practitioners committed to helping bring this vision into reality.

References

Carroll, M. (2014) *Effective Supervision for the Helping Professions*, 2nd edn. Sage Publications.

Hawkins, P. and Shohet, R. (2012) *Supervision in the Helping Professions*, 4th edn. Milton Keynes: O.U.P.

HCPC (2021) *Supervision.* Available online at: www.hcpc-uk.org/standards/meeting-our-standards/supervision-leadership-and-culture/supervision/ [Last accessed 10/12/23].

HCPC (2023) *Standards of Proficiency. Speech and Language Therapists.* Available online at: www.hcpc-uk.org/globalassets/resources/standards/standards-of-proficiency---speech-and-language-therapists.pdf [Last accessed: 04/12/23].

Health Education England (2020) *Workplace Supervision for Advanced Clinical Practice: An Integrated Multi-Professional Approach for Practitioner Development.*

Available online at: https://advanced-practice.hee.nhs.uk/workplace-supervision-for-advanced-clinical-practice-2/ [Last accessed on: 27/12/2023].

King, N., Bravington, A., Brooks, J., Hardy, B., Melvin, J. and Wilde, D. (2013) The Pictor technique: A method for exploring the experience of collaborative working. *Qualitative Health Research* 23, 1138–1152.

Royal College of Speech and Language Therapists (2017) *Information on Supervision.* Available online at: www.rcslt.org/members/delivering-quality-services/supervision/supervision-guidance/ [Last accessed: 04/12/2023.]

Royal College of Speech and Language Therapists (2023) *Professional Development Framework.* Available online via: https://www.rcslt.org/wp-content/uploads/2023/03/RCSLT-Professional-Development-Framework-2023.pdf [Last accessed: 27/12/2023].

Schuck, C. and Wood, J. (2011) *Inspiring Creative Supervision.* Jessica Kingsley Publishers

Stoltenberg, C. and Delworth, U. (1987) *Supervising Counsellors and Therapists.* San Francisco, CA: Jossey-Bass.

Stoltenberg, C., McNeil, B. and Delworth, U. (1998). *IDM Supervision: An Integrated Developmental Model for Supervising Counsellors and Therapists.* San Francisco: Jossey-Bass Publishers.

Wilson, P. and Long, I. (2008) *Big Book of Blobs.* Routledge.

Index